Talk, Think, Feel

Talk, Think, Feel

Perspectives of Doctors, Children with Cancer, and Their Families

Nathaniel Bayer

∞

TO PROGRESS

Contents

Foreword

"Childhood cancer is not happy kids with sweet shiny bald heads and brave smiles. Childhood cancer is not something that is given to kids because they are strong enough to handle it. Childhood cancer is not sunshine and love. Childhood cancer is scary. Childhood cancer is dark. Childhood cancer ruins families and lives. It is probably one of the most stressful, heart wrenching things in the world. The way childhood cancer is portrayed is not accurate."

—Maya Thompson

To conceptualize cancer or think about all its emotions is an individual process and one with complex intricacies that would take a lifetime to unravel. Cancer is a space with infinite paths towards understanding and experiencing. Each traveler must traverse his or her own route. This book explores the emotions of cancer from many perspectives, but its account is highly colored by my own experience as a medical student intending to specialize in pediatric oncology. Its limitations include that my vantage point was not developed as a pediatric oncologist, parent, family member, or child with cancer. It is neither a how-to book nor a clinical guide to those experiencing a loved one with cancer firsthand. It is, however, a portrayal of emotions in the field of pediatric oncology with careful thought and intent to spur further discourse and thought on the subject. So, if these emotional themes provoke human reactions, which I hope they will, I encourage you to talk with your family, friends, and healthcare providers. The value in this conversation is its continuation. Starting with this statement is not to discount my work, but to illuminate its foundation and provide insight into the way I portray cancer throughout the following book.

As I reflect on the components of my piece, I know some of Thompson's comments are relevant to my depiction. Yet, I stand by my thought process in portraying the emotions of cancer as a balance between positive and negative, and I recognize my slant towards positivity and optimism. I believe childhood cancer is currents of sunshine, hope, and love co-existing with themes of darkness, sadness, and pain. One set of feelings does not negate or denigrate the other. In both emotional undercurrents, we can find meaning and beauty. Her statement that "childhood cancer ruins families and lives" is only if we let it. As you continue to read, I hope you will form your own thoughts on the emotional makeup of childhood cancer.

Introduction

"When the Japanese mend broken objects, they aggrandize the damage by filling the cracks with gold. They believe that when something's suffered damage and has a history, it becomes more beautiful."

—Barbara Bloom

This book is a conversation about emotions and feelings. Its subject matter is children with cancer, but it is really an exploration of emotional themes examined through the lens of pediatric oncology. In oncology as in life, there exists a full spectrum of emotional experiences. Happiness, sadness, fear, anger, shock; they have all entered our own lives at certain points just as they have entered the lives of those touched by children with cancer. *Talk, Think, Feel: Perspectives of Doctors, Children with Cancer, and Their Families* provides the voices and perspectives of doctors, patients, families, and my own as a medical student on a topic we far too rarely discuss.

What follows is a collection of thoughts, stories, and observations of clinical encounters organized around discrete emotions. Each chapter is an analysis of one specific emotion or idea from multiple perspectives. The source material is

1

based largely on my two month cross-country tour of the United States in which I interviewed twenty pediatric oncologists at seven of the top major metropolitan children's hospitals and observed hundreds of clinical encounters while shadowing providers. I have included extensive direct quotes from the physicians to allow their own accounts and reflections to be presented unedited so that each is its own voice. Their narratives have been supplemented with my own thoughts. This book is based on doctor and patient stories about children's lives and even their deaths. All of them are factual, and in all of them, the raw truth is profound. To protect the privacy of doctors, patients, and hospitals, no identifying information is included and small details have been changed to ensure anonymity.

No matter what your connection is to children with cancer, I invite you to embark on this emotional exploration and find meaning within these pages. Some of you may have dealt with these emotions on a personal level in contexts similar to the ones described. I hope you will find comfort in reflecting on the commonalities and differences in your own story. For readers who may have no personal experience with pediatric cancers, I hope this book will serve to foster some understanding of the illness experience and its emotions, and to reflect on your own. Read the chapters in order or jump around creating an individualized path. Read the entire book or only one section depending on your objectives and emotional state.

As you read, I encourage you to think about the stories, the words, and the feelings. Consider how you might respond in the role of doctor, patient, or family member. Reflect upon the material, and share your reactions and sentiments. To feel is a remarkable gift. It is the characteristic that defines us as human. The splendor felt through positive emotions becomes unmatched in its glory when we are able to fully experience it. Even in its negative forms, feelings have beautiful meaning in spite of their sometimes painful reverberations.

It is my hope that you are able to talk, think, or feel even a bit more about emotions after reading this book. Fill your cracks with gold and find magnificence in their existence. Do not try to forget them, but experience your suffering as you experience your life—fully. In doing so, seek purpose and meaning. Find beauty in the emotional spectrum of your life, and then share it with the world in whatever way you can.

CHAPTER 1

Sadness
Doctors

"One day many years ago a man walked along and stood in the sound of the ocean on a cold sunless shore and said, "We need a voice to call across the water, to warn ships; I'll make one. I'll make a voice like all of time and all of the fog that ever was; I'll make a voice that is like an empty bed beside you all night long, and like an empty house when you open the door, and like trees in autumn with no leaves. A sound like the birds flying south, crying, and a sound like November wind and the sea on the hard, cold shore. I'll make a sound that's so alone that no one can miss it, that whoever hears it will weep in their souls, and hearths will seem warmer, and being inside will seem better to all who hear it in the distant towns. I'll make me a sound and an apparatus and they'll call it a Fog Horn and whoever hears it will know the sadness of eternity and the briefness of life."

The Fog Horn blew."

—Ray Bradbury, *The Fog Horn*

S adness is the deepest and lowest of emotions. Those in its throes often cannot see the path to happiness, for when sadness saturates a person's being his perspective becomes short, narrow, and dark. It leaves its

4

targets visibly wallowing, those who are near may share in the feeling, ignore its presence, or try to pull the affected from its grip. Sadness requires much dexterity to manage. While many assume this emotion pervades pediatric oncology, opinions from within the field largely disagree. Yes, sadness infuses many families and lives, but it can often be altered, ultimately making space for more positive emotions to take hold. Doctors share in moments or periods of sadness, but are able to navigate through with support. In permitting sadness to exist and by exploring it, we become more able to recognize and weaken its hold on ourselves and others—doctors, patients, and families alike.

Witnessing others' sadness has always been difficult, perhaps even more difficult than experiencing my own. I feel empty and powerless, yet simultaneously drawn to intervene. It's not that I enjoy situations where others are devastated, but in a simple way, I feel at home. I feel like it's where I'm supposed to be, helping patients and families navigate that emotional journey. In medicine, patients and colleagues experience sad and dark times with a need for someone to support and guide others forward. I hope to be one of those people guiding with hope, humor, love, dedication, and knowledge. I am learning strategies to be comfortable when close to sadness and am becoming more adept in addressing it. This will hopefully serve my future patients, families, and self well.

In gathering the material for this book, I interviewed twenty different pediatric oncologists across the United States. I asked about their opinions on the field with an emotional focus. I probed into their motivations and strategies in practice style, patient experiences, and word choice in encounters. One of my favorite questions to ask was how they respond to the assumption that a career in pediatric oncology "must be so sad". In their answers, I found clarification, perspective, and a surprise. A general theme that emerged was that treating children with cancer isn't actually all that sad. Most agreed that there are sad moments, but they asserted that the sheer privilege of being part of those moments and the happiness in the majority of children who are cured eclipses any sadness. Many expressed they were doing what they were meant to do. It was remarkable to see similarities in response to my questions about sadness when their personalities and backgrounds differed in so many other ways.

In reflecting on the assertion that pediatric oncology is a sad profession, one doctor offers his opinion on the happiness in the field, and provides a thoughtful professional and personal definition of success:

> Well, sometimes I don't say I'm a pediatric oncologist. Sometimes I say I'm a pediatrician. But, you're right; if you say to somebody in the lay public that you're a pediatric oncologist, almost everybody will say, "That's the worst job ever, it's so sad."... So, what I tell them I think is the truth; that... it has very bad days—when you have to give somebody bad news or a patient dies. But thankfully, there are many more happy days because more of our patients do well than don't.
>
> You also have to define success beyond life and death. If you take a family in the

worst moment of their life, and you help them understand what's going on, and make this medical issue more tolerable for them—[help] the child not be in pain, to go to school, and do as many normal activities as they can—then, to me..., that is a success. You should feel like you're doing something good for the child and family. It would be ridiculous to deny that there are very sad moments in this field, but I think it really is almost the opposite. [I]t can make you more appreciative for what you have and put your own problems in perspective. Maybe paradoxically, you're actually more grounded and happier than if you were not in the field.

Many doctors seemed to offer the high cure rate of children with cancer as a strong rebuttal to the claim of sadness:

My response is it's actually not that sad because of all kids, 80% are cured. To see families get the worst news of their entire lives and then to go through a long, hard and difficult process over the course of time, even a couple of years, to come out on the other side is what we want. A lot of families will reprioritize things and make good changes in their life and really treasure time. It's nice to see those 80% of families that do well.

In the same vein:

> I would say right now we cure more than
> 80% of our patients. The ones we don't
> cure teach me something new about life
> every single day. There's no question
> about that.

> I have little doubt that I'm doing what I
> was gifted to do... I think I am blessed
> in the sense that I have a job that I never
> get bored with.

And another doctor:

> I say, "Some days are better than
> others." People don't really want to
> know... [but if] they say, "Well, you
> know, what's it really like?" I'll say, "70%
> of kids with childhood cancer are cured.
> So, really, most days are good." And
> then I hope they sort of leave it there.

To choose a view that is positive is a masterful skill.
It dictates your perspective on the world. Interestingly, many
doctors offered comparisons with other fields to assert
pediatric oncology's own tendency away from sadness. This
is fascinating to think about—is the field less sad if there are
situations or other medical disciplines that are sadder? Many
pointed to adult oncology having poor survival rates in an
attempt to justify their statements. Data from the National
Institute of Health (NIH) shows that among adults with all
cancers, the 5-year survival rate is about 68% whereas in

children the rate approaches 81%. Is this evidence that pediatric oncology isn't sad?

One doctor seemed to think so:

> I tell them it's not sad. You [the writer] saw "Maggie" [with leukemia] in clinic yesterday. She is a delightful, charming girl who's going to be cured with relatively nontoxic therapy. If there weren't pediatric oncologists, she would already be dead.

> I think medical oncology is sad because so many patients die. Our cure rates are much higher and our patients can tolerate much more therapy. At the end of the day, they're still kids. Of course, it's sad and tragic when a child dies of anything, including cancer, but that is, fortunately in our field, not as common as in medical [adult] oncology.

> There are certainly days where I cry or go to my patients' funerals… but on the day to day I don't actually find it all that sad. I find it quite uplifting that we have effective therapies. Years ago, everyone uniformly died.

> I am quick to say, "It is not sad." It's sad when children die, but it would be sadder if people weren't there to help them.

This doctor offered a similar comparison to adult oncology:

> I say, "No, I don't find it that way." I can understand why people see it that way. Sometimes I distinguish it from adult oncology where I feel like they cure fewer patients. I get a lot of satisfaction out of… meeting someone [with a] grave disease [and] saying there's a cure. To walk them through that whole process is very gratifying. You [the writer] were on rounds with us this morning. It's not all doldrums. It's playing with some pretty cool, happy, and cute kids. Just helping them live in the moment and get through difficult therapy. I find that very fulfilling.

In this extended response below, there are many more comparisons. Here are her thoughts:

> It is absolutely not true. Yes, it can be sad, but medicine can always be sad, because medicine is not 100% successful so there are going to be plenty of failures, and the failures are sad. Is it sadder, the loss of a child than the loss of an adult? To a certain degree it is, because a child is the future and an adult is a little bit less. But to me, it is much more difficult to deal with the death of an adolescent than to deal with the death of a little one.

I think that the loss of a thirty-five-year-old mom with three kids is probably worse than the loss of a child. I don't know. It could be. I am not saying that one is better than the other or less.

But I don't think this is a sad field because the sadness of it is in your rational way of seeing them. If I see my clinic [as] kids with serious diseases, and some of them will not make it, yes, it is sad. But if I see my clinic as kids who came in quite sick and now are much better. Looking at them... they laugh and they play, and we think they have an ability to recover. It is amazing. It is not a sad environment.

It may be sad when you think about what the possibilities are, but when I actually work day by day, it is not sad to me. The majority of kids are cured. Part of it is related to the cancer diagnosis. Yes, there is a big component of unknown in cancer, but if I say that I am a neurologist is it any better? I think certain neurologic diseases are way worse than oncologic diseases. Or cardiac diseases, where they impair your life—for your entire life—are quite sad. Sickle cell disease is horrible. It doesn't have the stigma of cancer, but it is quite sad to see the "sicklers" come in screaming of pain a couple of times a year. They worry

> in their minds that [they can be in pain]
> at any time.
>
> So no, I don't see pediatric oncology as
> sad at all.

Some of the questions I had when thinking about the above pediatric oncologist's response included: How to quantify the level of sadness? Should it be determined by the length of life—"well she had a good, long life"—when talking about an older person? Or should it center on contributions—"he touched so many others' lives in his short time"? Does the manner of death—a tragic car accident or a prolonged degenerative disease—matter in the quantification of sadness? What is the saddest of all deaths? Is this even fair to compare?

Other responses were more about perspective and focusing on the happiness in even one encounter per day to sustain a positive outlook:

> I tell them it used to be a death sentence,
> but it's not the case anymore. We cure a
> lot of kids with leukemia. We certainly
> have a lot more work to do in terms of
> solid tumors. A lot of those kids we're
> curing only about 50 or 60%. That's a
> challenge.
>
> We also have a lot of success stories, and
> it's getting them to become a success
> story that keeps you going. That's the
> great thing about pediatrics and
> oncology; no matter how bad it gets,

there is always one kid who makes you laugh during the day. There's always one to put a smile on your face. And as long as that's the case, then you are fine. I think as long as I have that kid, that one kid who puts a smile on my face, then it's worth it. We tend to be "glass-half-full" type of people until there's no more reason to be. Yeah, that's what I tell them… we actually have a lot of success stories.

These are individuals who have much developed perspective and experience. Looking through the multitude of responses from these doctors, it becomes evident that they do not think this field is defined by its sadness. Rather, it is one filled with privilege, fulfillment, success, and appreciation. There are many vantage points in thinking about children with cancer. To characterize it as purely happy is false, but perhaps it is closer to "not sad" than "sad".

CHAPTER 2

Hope

"There is no medicine like hope, no incentive so great, and no tonic so powerful as expectation of something tomorrow."

—Orison Swett Marden

Hope sustains us. It is the best shield against misery and the strongest ally in our struggles and failures. It is a voice urging us to not give up no matter the challenge. Hope is perhaps the emotion that can most stand its ground when other emotions try to take hold. A person can be terrified, but if hopeful, can also be brave. A person can be devastated by circumstances, but if hopeful, can rebuild. A person can be weak, but if hopeful, can become strong. Cancer disrupts the normal structure and relationships in the lives of children and their families. It can deprive fathers from walking their daughters down the wedding aisle. It makes mothers wonder if they're still mothers if their only child passes away. It leaves siblings feeling neglected when their birthdays are overshadowed by their brother's cancer. Cancer takes an emotional toll on doctors inside and outside of the workplace. Its greed is insatiable. Yet, cancer cannot consume the hopes of doctors, families, and patients if they don't let it.

I am filled with hope as I enter my residency in pediatrics. I would define this feeling as an optimism that I will continue to develop my knowledge, connect with my patients, and fully explore the scientific and emotional frontiers of medicine. As a medical student, I have entered lives only briefly, albeit at great depth. A clinical rotation lasts six to eight weeks at most, often much less. Patient relationships are too short for many students to be fully aware of the clinical and psychosocial outcomes. Many students leave with a sense of uncertainty about the fate of their patients whom they don't see after the rotation ends. Despite this uncertainty, I was left with a feeling of such hope. While it may be overzealous positivity, I had strong feelings that my patients' illnesses would improve and that I had some beneficial role in their care. Perhaps I needed to tell myself that to persevere and not be consumed by negativity.

In my meeting doctors across the country and interviewing them on their motivations and emotions, I identified tremendous differences in personality, interests, practice styles, and communication methods. However, I observed a common thread in their expressions of hope. Some sustain it through religion, others define it through scientific progress, and many uphold it by focusing on patient successes.

Whatever their maintenance strategy, pediatric oncologists as a whole were quite hopeful. Perhaps the field attracts the hopeful or perhaps the field encourages it in its providers. Regardless, the communal emotion seems to reinforce itself and build within the healthcare team. It becomes part of the shared emotional experience of patients, families, and physicians. Fostering hope is one the most important objectives. In the words of one doctor:

> It's whether you look at life with the cup half-full or half-empty. There are patients we save who otherwise would never have had a chance. I hope by the end of my career that I bring something to the table that will significantly advance the field; but to get there, you can't sit outside. You've got to be in the field to advance the field.

Another doctor agreed with the half-full analogy, adding that perspective is important to maintain emotional strength:

> You don't get into this business if you're not going to be a hands-on type of manager of your patients. This just is not the right field for that. I always say as oncologists, we're kind of "half-glass-full-type" of people. So, the way I manage my emotions and my thought processes when a patient of mine is dying is that I try to look for the small victories. I take comfort in small victories. Can I get them to their Make a Wish Trip? You know, can I get them to their High School prom, can I make them comfortable? Those little things. Ultimately, I can't get them to a cure, I can't get them extra life, but I can at least make it as comfortable—their last few days or whatever—as pleasurable as

possible. If what makes them happy is going home and watching football with their father or something like that, we will make that happen. So I think, I take comfort in those little victories and I think I try to focus on those… rather than, you know…

There is a choice in perspective throughout pediatric oncology. The ability to control emotions by consciously deciding to be hopeful or by choosing to be happy is such an important skill, especially when dealing with cancer on a daily basis. In a single day, a doctor may tell a new patient they have cancer, plan to discharge a child for hospice care, and perform a procedure showing a patient is in remission or relapse. This emotional rollercoaster requires great control and thoughtfulness to navigate. Doctors need to effectively and compassionately provide the best medical care while fostering hope in patients, families, the care team, and themselves. For this task, it seems that they might have to be exceptionally hopeful.

Physicians do not suspend reality in their outlooks for their patients, but rather choose to remain hopeful. It's easy to be hopeful when discussing a "good" case of leukemia, a type of blood cancer with over a 90% rate of cure. But even with some difficult brain tumors where the chance of cure is less than 10%, doctors still maintain this optimism. Some are quite introspective in recognizing this quality in themselves. Here's one such optimist:

Part of the reason that I can continue doing this job is because I believe that there is someone who makes up the

10%. And maybe my patient is going to be in that 10% who survives. I think if you don't have that belief, when you do have these kids that have horrible prognoses, it makes it hard to get up out of bed and do your job every day. I think having that kind of outlook is important.

The desire for a miracle for a patient in the 10% can still exist even in the face of the statistical probabilities:

As a physician, I want all of my patients to live. I hope against hope for the miracle that their parents hope for too. Even though, rationally, I know that it probably isn't going to come for a lot of my patients.

Sometimes doctors are too hopeful. They may be viewed as being too aggressive with treatment; too optimistic or too desperate that their last ditch efforts on the fringe of scientific reason may work. It is critical for physicians to recognize that while patients and families do not always understand many of the medical intricacies of cancer treatment, they are incredibly perceptive to identify hope in a physician. If a physician displays too much hope—if there is such a thing—then patients, especially at the "end", may choose treatment courses they otherwise would not have chosen.

Here is one physician's story illustrating this point. It is about a fifteen-year-old boy with advanced thymic carcinoma, a solid cancer of the thymus organ in the upper chest. The patient's tumor hadn't responded to multiple chemotherapy trials, and the physician was considering a last ditch effort to try cetuximab, another chemotherapy agent:

> This was the thymic carcinoma kid, actually. And the drug was cetuximab which has been shown to have some effect on thymoma, which is a different disease from thymic carcinoma. But, there is a little bit of overlap.

> There isn't a lot of data in regard to cetuximab and thymic carcinoma per se, but because there was a little bit of overlap I thought it could work. You know, it was worth a shot. But I think at that point, he... I mean I'd thrown the kitchen sink at him, and you know we had been treating him a long time, so at that point it was clear that he was tired and he didn't want anymore. It was incumbent upon me to recognize that.

> Sometimes I have to stop myself and ask, "Am I treating myself?" This drug may have potentially benefited this patient. Perhaps I was pushing it a little bit, but this patient had been through a lot already and he had been through multiple, multiple courses of chemotherapy. It always came back. It was coming back really strong, and I thought, "Oh maybe this will work for him". After talking it over with him, he made clear to me that he didn't want

anymore. I found myself having to hold
myself back from pushing this, from
pushing this drug. Because I said, "Am I
doing it for him or am I doing it for
myself?" You know, ultimately I think I
got to the point where I was comfortable
with what he really wanted and so he
went home, and we ended up not giving
him the drug. It was a long shot
admittedly. Did I really think it was going
to cure him? No, no. But as doctors, I
think we are in the business of offering
what we can. We're not in the business
of really saying no, right? So, I think
sometimes I have to check myself and
find out, and really kind of listen to the
patient and determine what is it that they
truly want?

In partnering with patients and families, hope is
strongly encouraged at the beginning of diagnoses. In
pediatric cancers, the initial treatment goal for almost all
cases is to attempt to cure the cancer. So, it is easy to portray
hope at the beginning of a new diagnosis and to support
families at that point because, as one doctor put it, "People
are generally hopeful, they want to live. I can't think of any
patients or families, even teenagers, who have said, 'Okay,
well just let me go.' " When sharing a new diagnosis of
cancer with a patient, physicians infuse their messages with
abundant hope:

> Anytime you're giving something bad
> like that [a cancer diagnosis], try to give
> them some sense of hope also. There are

very few diagnoses we deal with nowadays that you can't give some level of hope... There's always some good thing that you can present to the family. Like we can figure out what exactly his diagnosis is and we will have a plan to treat this. Our goal for treatment is a cure.

Another physician portrayed nearly the same sentiment:

Always have some sort of message of hope that counters your gloom-and-doom, "You have cancer". I think that that has always been something that I've weaved into the conversation as well. "Your child has this," or "You have this cancer, but we can do something about it. This is what we can do." For me as a physician and also, I like to think, for the families... that giving them a plan and some course of action... that it makes it somewhat easier.

Even when the initial diagnosis is one of the "bad" types of cancer with a poor prognosis, physicians agree that instilling hope is sometimes the most important goal in these initial conversations:

We usually try, even if you know the outcome is not so great, you usually always have to leave with a note of optimism and a note of... make them feel that they are in a place where there is

experience, where the care of the child is
very comprehensive, and where
everything will be done to achieve the
best outcome possible.

You usually leave with a note of
optimism, but also at the same time a
realistic approach. Because usually, it is
normal that what they will retain is
actually your optimism.

So you don't want them to get a false
idea. You are a little bit realistic with
some optimism because you also know
that there is time for many, many more
conversations afterwards.

All physicians I interviewed seemed to agree on this idea. At
the beginning, they tend to be upfront about diagnosis and
treatment plan while employing a looser strategy when it
comes to being completely upfront about prognosis. While
still maintaining honesty, they frame the discussion regarding
prognosis to maximize hope with parents and older children.

Prognosis is explained to patients and families as a
narrative, not numbers. Almost all doctors seemed to be
uncomfortable using numbers or percentages for prognosis
in the early conversations. While the scientific literature and
medical studies have published percentages for most
pediatric cancers, such as a 90% 5-year survival rate for
children with Wilms tumors, these numbers can be very
confusing, hard to interpret, and depressing for patients and
families. Statistics are often counter-productive to instilling a
sense of hope.

As one physician commented:

> Regarding prognosis, I don't often say
> the percentages unless I'm directly asked.
> Because at least in my way of thinking,
> again if the percentage is 30%, you don't
> have a test that can figure out if he is on
> the 30 or the 70 side of that. There's no
> way to answer that.
>
> I think most families need to know if
> there's hope or not. At diagnosis, there's
> never no hope. Especially at a place like
> this; there's always something new to try.

Doctors seem even less likely to be upfront about prognosis
when they are directly talking with the child who has cancer:

> When I talk with the child, I am upfront
> about the name of the disease and that
> it's a type of cancer. I talk about the
> proposed treatment. I tend to not talk
> about prognosis early on with the child
> because our initial default for almost all
> patients is that we will treat them in
> some way with anti-cancer therapy and
> hope for a good response even if
> statistically their likelihood of cure is low.
> We will still initiate anti-cancer therapy
> with the hope that they are one of the
> few who survive and beat the odds, or at
> least that they'll have palliation and
> prolongation of their life with a
> reasonable quality of life.

All of these strategies are aimed to create hope for patients and families at the initial time of diagnosis. Most people seem to easily identify and grasp onto this emotion at the beginning perhaps out of an instinctual emotional survival mechanism. As shattering as the news of a cancer diagnosis, if patients and families have even a speck of hope, they can march forward. Doctors need parents to be like this mother of a three-month-old little girl who was, "taking this in intellectually really amazingly". The mother's hope was so strong even though her beloved daughter was in the neonatal intensive care unit (NICU) because she was found to have a type of blood cancer and couldn't breathe on her own. In the darkest times, she found hope. She would compassionately look upon her new baby girl hooked up to a breathing machine with tubes and monitoring devices covering almost every inch of her tiny body. She maintained a positive outlook despite facing everything alone as her husband was in the military and deployed overseas. I remember her saying, "She's in it to win and so are we," a simple and beautiful assertion of hope's power in a mother.

In these situations, parents just knowing that there's a possibility that their child will survive is enough to sustain that sliver of hope. In one family, all it took was reassurance. This was a family where the sixteen-year-old son had just been diagnosed with acute myelogenous leukemia (AML). He came into the hospital because of recent vomiting and neck pain. After spending a week in the hospital getting initial chemotherapy, he started to have belly pain and diarrhea. Overnight, he went into septic shock, meaning his blood pressure had dropped to dangerously low levels because of a systemic infection. He was rushed to the intensive care unit (ICU) and intubated because he couldn't breathe on his own. He was hooked up to monitors, was unconscious, and his toes had turned black from the lack of oxygen and blood flow. His father, distraught and lost in this blur, needed answers, "Given the situation, can his body withstand this?" Recognizing that this father needed hope, his doctor responded, "Children have recovered from this point. Absolutely I've seen kids recover from where he is." This simple reassurance was a powerful infusion of hope. In pediatric oncology, parents face similar situations like this and really need hope to remain emotionally grounded. While the dad's emotional state is unlikely to change the outcome for his son, the doctor felt the statement was needed at that very moment. Was it more to offer momentary solace or was it the real truth? This child may likely be on the road towards death, but the doctor chose not to have that conversation. She chose to prioritize hope in that instance.

Often, children have their own ways of maintaining hope. It's remarkable to watch them when they are in the room with parents and doctors talking about either their cancer or prognosis. They have a mechanism of selective listening and not absorbing information that is too overwhelming or negative. At some point, children shut off emotionally despite being physically present. In my experience, this self-preservation strategy occurs primarily in those aged six to twelve. Here's one physician's reflection on talking about bad news with children in the room:

> I think that it's important to include them, and I never kick the kids out of the room for any of these discussions. What I've noticed is that children very often, they will sort of shut down. They'll stop listening when it gets too much for them. They are very good at

that… When I'm in talking to families, giving them bad news… the kids will be involved and as soon as you start moving towards bad things they'll start playing.

Doctors give hope as in the situation above, but sometimes they have to take it away or temper its level. Through observing many interactions between providers, patients, and families, I've identified hope as a prevalent theme in these discussions. In most of these conversations, the amount of hope encouraged was managed with great care and compassion. But in some, it seemed doctors let false hope grow too strong or they hastily crushed it without fully exploring its context. For although patients "do better when [they] know what the score is", the way they are informed can have great consequences in breaking trust and causing despair.

Patients remember when doctors tell them statements with a negative connotation as in things they can't or won't be able to do. A fourteen-year-old girl most remembers this about her cancer treatment: "All the no's that I couldn't do. I couldn't go back to school, I couldn't play softball, and I couldn't eat what I wanted. 97% of my body was cancer. If I had waited another day, I would have died." While this may be a dramatic perspective of an adolescent, it describes her feeling like she has lost the authority that is so important to developing an identity. Her thoughts illustrate that patients remember each of these conversations about what they cannot do and cannot be. This vignette reminds us that there is a choice in presenting situations and establishing plans. It is best to frame conversations and allocate emotions in a positive light with a conscious manner. We must remember to save a place for hope when we are constructing our conversations and navigating situations.

I remember one such situation where the doctor seemed to take away hope prematurely without adequately refocusing it. This was a nine-year-old boy who had been diagnosed with retinoblastoma, a tumor of the eye, when he was just four months old and was left nearly blind after completing the treatment. He was brought in to clinic for a follow-up visit where he completed an electroretinography, a sophisticated vision test. At that visit, this discussion occurred:

> Dad: How well are his retinas working?

> Doctor: So far, his retinas are working very well. But with retinoblastoma, his vision is now bad.

> Dad: There's no way to improve it?

> Doctor: Hopefully, we killed the tumor, but we can't bring back the retina.

> Dad: Well, he started completely blind. But now at least he can see and run.

> Doctor: That's good.

> Dad: He wants to become a doctor, but if he's blind, he can't be a doctor, right?

> Doctor: There are no medical schools with Braille. There are few medical

schools that would accept someone who they know is blind.

Dad: Yes.

Doctor: We're all done, and we got good information.

As the doctors and I left the room, I could see both the child and father crying a little as they thanked us for "our time". To me, that room felt so cold, still and somber as we walked out. It felt hopeless. I hated that feeling and promised to myself that I would try to never create it. I wished that this conversation had shifted to redefine and refocus hope in this father and child. While it is true that this boy could likely never become a doctor, to me, the way the doctor made the statement was too harsh and unforgiving. The doctor could have continued the conversation to further explore the dad's question and refocus the goal towards wanting a happy, healthy, and long life. He could have reminded and reassured the father and son that blind people can go to college and have successful careers in many fields. "No" can be one of the most challenging statements to deliver in a compassionate manner. That conversation became centered on what this boy couldn't do instead of what he can and will be able to do. These may seem like nuanced points of word choice and professional honesty, yet I believe that words and emotions are far more powerful than a lot of doctors and even patients realize. As Dr. Sara Murray Jordan says, "In medicine, as in statecraft and propaganda, words are sometimes the most powerful drugs we can use."

In difficult discussions such as above, it is important to leave a vestige of hope intact so that it can be built upon.

Doctors need to define and temper hope, not take it away. They may need to change hope's direction with patients and families. This emotion is crucial when the hope is for a cure, a "normal" life, or for one more meaningful experience before death. Along the whole course of treating children with cancer, hope needs to be cultivated. At some points it needs to be trimmed back, other times supported with stakes and fertilizer, and sometimes even uprooted and transplanted to a different setting. How to best grow hope is often determined by the doctors.

Even at the end of life, when care is being transitioned to non-curative options, one physician states:

> You don't want to take away hope. I think you can still say, "We're doing everything we can, we want you to know that... but with how sick you are... what's important to you? What are you hoping for? What would make today a good day? Let's just focus on that and the here and now."

This refocusing of perspective and hope is paramount when transitioning from attempting to cure the child of cancer to non-curative therapy. It is often done in concert with increasing the prioritization of comfort in the treatment plan. The care often involves palliative care providers, individuals who are masters in navigating hope, pain control, and emotions through these situations. This field of medicine has many misconceptions including that it is analogous to hospice, that it is "giving up" or "doing nothing", and that it is only useful when someone is dying.

All of these assumptions are incorrect. According to the Center to Advance Palliative Care:

> Palliative care is specialized medical care for people with serious illnesses. It is focused on providing patients with relief from the symptoms, pain, and stress of a serious illness—whatever the diagnosis. The goal is to improve quality of life for both the patient and the family. Palliative care is provided by a team of doctors, nurses, and other specialists who work together with a patient's other doctors to provide an extra layer of support. It is appropriate at any age and at any stage in a serious illness and can be provided along with curative treatment.

Just as hope needs to be supported from day one, so does palliative care. As one doctor states:

> The data show that families have dual goals. They have a cancer directed goal and they have a comfort directed goal. They shouldn't be looked at individually because people want us to do the very best we possibly can in terms of the cancer. They want to work towards cure but they also want to make sure that we're fighting for comfort right from the beginning. We think about palliative care as including that part of it, the comfort part of it, and the quality of life aspects.

Palliative care for any patient needs to be integrated from the first day. That doesn't mean that it should be a quality of life service consult or palliative care consult. It means that we as oncology providers need to integrate palliative care from the first day that someone comes in. We talk so much about palliative care concepts, concepts of relationship building from the very beginning, concepts of focusing on what the family's needs are, and expert communication skills, all of that is palliative care.

Palliative care really needs to be integrated from the first day. It shouldn't be seen as a specific phase. A lot of people talk about the palliative phase of life but really palliative care needs and issues should be integrated at all phases of the cancer trajectory and in all of the different stages. It just looks differently at each point.

Even in the field of palliative care where a large focus is on helping patients die with grace and in comfort, providers feel their field is defined by hope. Here's one physician on finding that perspective:

No. I'm not sad at all in the field. I would say hopeful. I would say even in my field of palliative care, hope sustains us. I would say that it's all about the perspective that you look at things. Yeah, if you're removed from the field it looks sad, but once in you're in the middle of the field, you recognize that it's really about hope.

I'm thinking about a good word... maybe compassion is a great word. Hope and compassion. Compassion I mean is to suffer with. Even though you are going through difficult times that may be sad for the family, you may be suffering with that family, you can hopefully remain hopeful. Yeah, I think those would be better assessments, compassion and hope.

The world of pediatric oncology can be emotionally devastating. Providers may lose their perspective when faced with the loss of a patient. Families can be torn apart by stress, sadness, and exhaustion. Children with cancer may question their identities as they deal with issues of life and death much earlier than their peers. These struggles are real, painful, and challenging. They require an incredible amount of conscious thought and reflection by all involved to persevere and maintain emotional stability. Hope is the strongest partner to support positivity and forward thinking. Hope is the strongest weapon in battling negativity and emotional ruin. Hope's power is great, its necessity for success is paramount, and its presence or lack thereof should never be overlooked in life and definitely not in children with cancer. If its importance is forgotten, all those involved will suffer: doctors, families, and patients. That is certainly something to be afraid of.

CHAPTER 3

Fear

"Fear imprisons… fear paralyzes… fear disheartens… fear sickens… fear makes useless…"

—Harry Emerson Fosdick

Fear is the most possessive of emotions. Its presence overwhelms the consciousness and prevents other more positive emotions—faith, hope, determination, and trust—from being felt by those it affects. When a person is fearful, his forward-thinking thought process becomes paralyzed. It is a state of darkness, worry, and panic with no apparent end in sight or direction to turn for help. Fear casts its shadow throughout the world of medicine, certainly in pediatric cancer. It looms over doctors, patients, and families. Addressing it requires knowing where to look.

For me as a medical student, there was the fear of saying the wrong thing to patients and families. I felt an enormous responsibility to perform perfectly, to say the right words, and to know the correct answers to questions. It was not so much the fear of making a medical error; it is almost impossible to compromise care or patient safety as a medical student. There are so many safeguards—residents, nurses, and supervising doctors—in place to double-check my orders and clinical work. However, words spoken to a family are final; they cannot be redacted or adjusted by a supervising doctor. They cannot be forgotten or undone. I remember one family who came in to the children's hospital late at night with their six-year-old son. He had been having daytime wetting accidents and difficulty starting his urinary stream, which were both unusual for him. His family doctor had diagnosed a urinary tract infection, sent him home with antibiotics, and ordered a follow-up ultrasound scan. When he completed the imaging five days later, it showed a five centimeter mass compressing his bladder. From the office, his family was told to go home, pack their belongings, and then head to the hospital. So, there they were in the hospital room at ten o'clock in the evening about to hear some of the worst news of their lives.

When a child comes in with a suspected cancer diagnosis, the fear is always palpable. It exudes from the parents in awkward glances, clenched fists, and nervous hand-holding. Their fear is most obvious by a look in their terrified eyes that I can only describe as unsettling. It is as if their eyes are realizing ahead of their brains that a cancer diagnosis is about to enter their otherwise ordinary lives. It is in those first moments talking to new families that I was most afraid. I felt unequipped by myself to respond, address, and console the parents and patient should they realize the diagnosis was cancer. Sometimes the team is almost certain of the cancer diagnosis from the preliminary tests, but we wait for the final results to confirm our suspicion and have a full family discussion. That way we can gather all the information and share the cancer diagnosis when the most senior doctor, the attending, is present. Often a medical student and a junior resident interview the new patient and family first when they arrive at the hospital. That situation is exactly what I remember with that boy and his family; the medical team knew ahead of time this was most likely cancer. I remember interviewing this boy's parents, painstakingly asking about their son's allergies, school, and family history of cancer. I remember interviewing the little boy, who was—as is usually the case—distractedly playing games, thoroughly confused by being in the hospital, and naïvely happy to be among so many people focused on him. I feared that by asking almost too carefully constructed questions and by tiptoeing around the word "cancer", that my compassionate, calm manner was a silent confirmation of their son's diagnosis. I was afraid I would say cancer instead of mass with a slip of my tongue. I was afraid of accidentally confirming a cancer diagnosis and opening the emotional floodgates without the seasoned senior doctor there to respond to the situation. However, the thing I feared most in this brief first encounter was that they would ask if their son had cancer. Thankfully, they didn't.

Each time I encountered a family at the beginning of their child's cancer journey, I became progressively more comfortable in that first interview. That fear of incorrectly choosing words gradually diminished in successive encounters. For me, in this situation, the solution to fear was experience. Yet, experience brings about its own set of fears within doctors. Sometimes knowing more does not mean becoming less afraid. Here are a physician's thoughts on that different but very real level of fear and concern:

> When it is a first diagnosis, it touches you because you see the reaction of the families, the child, and you know what is behind this thing: the diagnosis. You know a lot of things that can happen that

they don't know. You are trying to tell
them that it is hard, but we will get
through this and the outcome may be
good. But, you also know that even in
the best diagnosis you can get a
complication and be dead in two weeks.
You know a lot of things they don't
know, and so you have a different degree
of concern. But at the same time, you
obviously have a different degree of
emotional involvement.

Each person fears different outcomes because of this
knowledge gap between doctors and patients. While bridging
attempts are made with teaching and counseling parents and
children, the gap will always remain. Doctors train at length
and have seen thousands of patients before they practice
independently. This means that doctors are aware of all the
bad possibilities. They have seen their worst fears come true
in children with cancer, even in the ones with the best
prognoses. They have seen overwhelming infections quickly
cause life threatening sepsis and allergic reactions to standard
chemotherapeutic agents cause anaphylactic shock. With
each permutation of rare outcomes as personal experience, the
fear provoking possibilities in a new cancer diagnosis remain
real and alarming for physicians. In many cases, these fears
remain silent; doctors refrain from sharing their concerns
with patients or families because to do so would be to
completely overwhelm them. To admit them to other
providers would be to acknowledge their own fears of
vulnerability and of the unknown illness course.

From the doctors I interviewed across the country
and from my own experience with hundreds of doctor

trainees, we all seem to fear failing. The profession attracts some of the most accomplished, intelligent, and driven individuals. In the stakes of children with cancer, failing can instill a great sense of guilt. In one physician who treats cancer, failure is not just defined as death but is much broader:

> I think, at least for me, what is hard is mostly there is a sense of failure when something goes bad, when there is a relapse or you can't achieve another remission, you can't make them better. There is really a sense of failure, of frustration, and of everything you try not making any difference. It is sort of exasperating, like something needs to be done, a surgery needs to be done, or really there needs to be some sort of advancement... For me, it is really mostly a sense of failure...

> It is almost to a level of guilt like you were not able to achieve what you really wanted: to make them comfortable. This can be not only in the sense of cure but even at a point where everybody accepts palliation. Even the inability to achieve a certain level of comfort, a certain level of quality of life, it is quite disturbing.

> You may have accepted the fact that somebody may die, but the fact of not being able to allow them to die with dignity, it's as upsetting, frustrating, and

guilt building as if they were in therapy.
The way they leave the world is very,
very, very important for a lot of things.
For the kid and for the way the family
will remember the experience.

Doctors make choices. In the case of kids with
cancer, these choices culminate into continued life or death,
with varying level of comfort if the child is dying. Certain
poor outcomes make doctors feel a strong sense of personal
failure even if the choices made were in agreement with the
best standard of care. Doctors attempt to rationalize this
sense of failure to diminish its impact; they distance
themselves and their actions from that of the disease. It is
one answer to their fear of personal failure:

You know, you just kind of tuck it away.
Part of me knows that this is just the way
it is. I'm not the cause... I'm only doing
what I know how to do to help cure the
disease. If the disease comes back, it's
not my fault. It's the disease, it not
anyone's fault, it's the disease.

Cancer is not always curable. Furthermore, it is not as simple
as one choice resulting in a good or bad outcome, it is many
decisions and development over the course of the illness.
The specific chemotherapeutic drugs chosen, the early
introduction of an antibiotic, a successful or unsuccessful
pain regimen at the end of life, all of these will have different
patient consequences. Thus, there can be tremendous doubt
as the physician looks back on the treatment course. Some of
the outcomes will be poor, some patients will struggle, and
some will die; some may even die in what the physician

above deems as without "a certain level of comfort". This is perhaps the most distressing environment in pediatric oncology: to be part of a treatment team caring for a child who is struggling in pain or anguish in his or her last days or weeks. It is one of the most upsetting and guilt-inducing situations for a physician to be in.

Doctors seem to be fearful not only at the beginning when identifying the specific type of cancer diagnosis present, but also at checkpoints along the treatment course. In the field of pediatric cancer, we perform tests to see if our therapy is successful or if the cancer has continued growing despite treatment. Tests include imaging to see if the tumor has decreased in size or if any new tumors have grown, blood tests to determine if any cancer cells are in the blood, and procedures to take marrow out of the bones to check if the cancer is there. At each checkpoint and test, there is a possibility of both a good and bad result. Hence, these tests tend to create much fear for doctors, patients, and families alike. One oncologist speaks of this common fear between the families and herself:

> You do go through pretty much the same thing as families do, but maybe not to the same extent... I am fearful every time somebody has a surveillance scan, bone marrow, or CBC [Complete Blood Count, a blood test to check for cancer recurrence] the same way that a family would. I go through the same thing.

She speaks of the commonality of the fear of test results. In parents, this anticipation can create huge amounts of fright that disrupt their daily activities. One dad told me that he becomes so scared that he cannot sleep for the one month before the follow-up scans for his nine-year-old son with bilateral retinoblastoma, a type of eye cancer. The immense emotional buildup to these scans is a common one and one which hovers over parents, weighing down their spirits for long periods of time. It is one which culminates in either an explosion of happiness if the test result is good or a sinking devastation if the test result is bad. This can be a draining cycle as these tests occur every couple of months during active treatment and can continue almost annually for years after the end of active treatment.

Medicine is often not clear-cut. Difficult situations arise when test results aren't clear. The unknown of an ambiguous result comes with its own unique set of concerns, all of which are difficult to grasp for both providers and patients. A test with no clear results can spur distrust, disbelief, and denial. Modern medicine appears so binary to the public — either you have cancer or you do not, either the chemotherapy works or it does not — but in reality it is much more complex. Every test and every result has the small possibility of being indeterminate or incorrect. Thus, in rare settings where the scan showed no cancer, there may actually be cancer.

In one exchange below, there is such a sense of discomfort on both sides as a parent and doctor discuss such an ambiguous test result. The patient is an eighteen-year-old male with a high-risk pre-B cell ALL, a type of leukemia. He had a brain magnetic resonance imaging (MRI) scan to check if the leukemia had entered his brain or central nervous system.

This is the discussion of the results; it occurred while looking at the images of his brain on the computer:

> Doctor: The MRI showed this tiny little spot that we wanted to talk to you about. No one can say what it is. All that needs to be done is for it to be watched. You can tell this is really, really small. But it is brighter than it should be. No one can say what that is. We talked to everyone about it.
>
> Dad: Now what makes one spot lighter or darker?
>
> Doctor: When [he] got this, [he] got contrast and it means this spot takes up more. The plan will be to observe with MRIs.
>
> Dad: I don't want to worry.
>
> Doctor: It's thought to be an incidental finding. I don't know what to tell you.
>
> Dad: Ok.

What is implicit in this conversation is that the "bright spot" might be cancer; it may have spread to a location in the brain. If it did, it would absorb more contrast dye which appears white when imaged with an MRI. This is different than normal brain tissue which appears more gray or dark on a scan. This is why doctors call it "bright". The other possibility is that this child's brain is just structured that way and the bright spot means nothing; the aberrant finding was always present, but was only found because we took an image of it. In fancy doctor words, it is "incidental", as the doctor states. Either way, this unknown presents a unique type of fear. The conversation is steeped in the doctor' language of hedging as he refers to the "bright" spot as "incidental", qualifying with "thought to be" and emphasizing its size as "really, really small" in an attempt to comfort the father. After all, the doctor does not "know what to tell [them]". Interestingly, this discussion quickly pivoted to talking about feeling better in time to get the young man home for his senior ball, a topic much easier to talk about. As they chatted about cummerbunds and tuxedo rentals, it seemed they almost forgot about the scan results from a moment before. More likely, this uncertainty was scary for both parties, so they both decided not to dwell on that fear anymore.

For children with cancer, fear can mangle their identity and development manifesting in sadness, anger, depression, or distancing. Children may be unable to vocalize or understand their fears or they may submerge their fears in order to protect their parents. To see a child with cancer in fear is a harrowing experience; it shames and puts into perspective your own fears and worries. I am filled with awe for these children for their bravery against fears that I cannot fully comprehend in magnitude or sentiment. One doctor, reflecting on her experience in oncology and palliative care, remarked that children's fears are the same as those of adults. They "always revolve around the issues of pain and separation".

The fear of pain is universal in children. If they are cognizant of an upcoming procedure, they must be constantly reassured "that the procedure is done under anesthesia, they won't feel anything, and to expect that. For them, it is a fear thing." Some, like an eight-year-old boy with relapsed ALL experiencing a pain crisis, have so much pain that they are afraid to even move or sit up on the commode. His particular situation was complicated because he was enrolled in a Phase I trial of a treatment drug called MLN. This drug had no chance of curing him and only a slight chance of prolonging his life. Yet the trial's enrollment criteria stipulated that participants could not be on a patient controlled analgesic (PCA), a type of pain medication delivered continuously and whenever the patient pushes a button. The patient's current pain regimen, Dilaudid every four hours and a long-acting Fentanyl patch, both morphine analogues, was not working. His doctor was in a difficult position. When should the patient be withdrawn from the trial so that a different pain management strategy could be implemented?

The fear of physical pain is relatable; we all appreciate what it means to be afraid of that kind of pain. For the most part, doctors can lessen that fear with reassurance and by using effective modern pain medications. Says a physician:

> The pain we can [manage] with a great deal of certainty. [We can] say, "We will do everything so that you will be comfortable. If you ever feel that we aren't giving you enough medicine then you can tell us. We can give you more because being comfortable is something we can do."

But the fear that is more emotional or more related to identity or death is harder to grasp and address. These fears are universal in pediatric cancer, although they tend to manifest differently in younger versus older children.

While a three year old girl's understanding of being neutropenic is certainly limited, her fear when her protective face mask was removed was immense. Being neutropenic means that the immune cells in your body are low; you are at much higher risk of getting an infection. In our patients whose chemotherapy has caused them to have no white blood cells to fight infections, they are at a high risk when surrounded by others' germs. To protect themselves, they wear face masks that cover their mouths and noses so they cannot inhale others' germs. This little girl, bald and clad in pink pajamas with a white face mask, would scream at the top of her lungs, "I'm neutropenic! I'm neutropenic!" whenever her mask was touched or moved by anyone, especially the doctor to examine the inside of her mouth which required removal of the mask. She had come to believe that this mask powerfully protected her, and she was so afraid to lose its shield even for a moment. Whether she was afraid of an infection or death or was mirroring her mother's fear concerning that mask remains unclear.

Like pain, separation induces fear. Separation can be from people and relationships, but the ultimate separation is death. In pediatric oncology, many patients have long lives; other patients die of their disease. When this latter outcome happens, the doctors, parents, and child each become aware that the cancer has become incurable. While the timeline for this recognition and cognitive processing is very different for each involved, the path leading to a child's death from cancer is one filled with raw emotion and much fear for all. It is one which many physicians I interviewed have called an "honor" to participate in. To navigate death with children and families is both a daunting and humbling responsibility. One young fellow at the beginning of her career wondered, "How do you make death less scary?" In its sheer enormity, this question is profound. It begs for an answer.

According to another oncologist, children understand the idea of separation:

> They will say things like "I'm going to miss mommy and daddy, they're going to miss me. Will they be okay without me?" So, oftentimes kids just need that reassurance... That's again, what does everybody want? Everybody wants the two most primitive things. They don't want to hurt and they want to feel like if there's a separation, there's a place they're going and there's a place where they'll be remembered because kids will, I mean a lot of people but mostly kids, will say things like, "Are you going to keep my pictures on the wall? Are you going to keep my pictures in the album? Are you going to do this, that, or the other thing?"

Children seek reassurance that they will not be forgotten or impermanent. It is a fear of profound anguish. A seven-year-old boy worries that his parents will throw out the photo albums and forget him after he passes away. In the imaginative mind of a child, this can be the thought process. One social worker had this to say about how her hospital addresses this theme of remembrance to help both children and parents:

> Give them something they can take with them forever. I think that one of the things that definitely we do great here but I think most children's hospitals do. When the children are [near] the end of life, not doing well the whole team from the nurses and the chaplains, and the Child Life worker they sort of get together and put together remembrance boxes. They do handprints for the children and do Plaster of Paris molds of the children's hand and all these things like that. Give the parents things to take with them. It is the memory in thing, but they can try to remember some good things

> We have everywhere in the hospital all these amazing pictures of kids. We have amazing photographers and they will get the photographer there and take pictures of parents and their children. You're able to support the family. Try to make even this horrible moment something that they can take away something from

Some families are so lost in grief and emotion that their rational thought is fragmented. This presents significant challenges, as a child's death requires much planning. Few parents have experience in organizing this process with their child, so they need assistance with these details. Large teams of doctors, nurses, social workers, and counselors are immensely helpful in supporting parents and families through the process. One of these details is place—the location where parents wish their child to be when he or she dies:

> Most parents say that kids always are happier at home. Some parents acknowledge being scared that they're not going to be able to manage and so we always try to say we can start off at home if it gets to be too much we'll bring you in. Then a lot also depends upon the resources we have in the community. So if they live nearby and have a good pediatric hospice or home care, then we're more confident and try to keep them home.

The way that children process fear at the end of their lives is both heartbreaking and captivating to witness in its humanity and beauty. Fear can be expressed through many emotions including regret, hope, faith, and rarely anger. One doctor states:

> I think anger is in a minority of people. I think there's some anger. I think there are people who would say they're angry at God or angry at whatever it is or angry at this situation but most people aren't angry. Most people... almost everybody is angry at the scenario or some aspect during their treatment. They may be angry that their child is so sick. But anger

as an ongoing issue not something we
seem to find much actually.

Some children process their fears into regrets. Older
children, teenager lament that they will never get
married, have their own children, or graduate. Younger
children are fearful of what will happen to their stuff. All are
afraid it will hurt. All are afraid to be alone. Some kids "may
never bring up the D word" even if they have thought about
it. Kids are remarkable in reading situations and putting
together the pieces as they start to feel sicker. That is why
one oncologist has these tough conversations even with
young kids.

> When I think death seems more
> imminent, we have a separate
> conversation [where we talk about the
> idea that] we think that you're going to
> die of your cancer. Often even young
> kids have some experience with death in
> the family and exploring that "Do you
> know what death is

> I would try to use the word death or die,
> but frame it as well and say. You might
> not know what that means or what that
> is like. Let me tell you. The words
> everyone uses, falling asleep and not
> waking up?" Depending on religious
> beliefs or whatever is going to happen,
> seeing other people who've died, and
> things like that, but trying to make it as
> not scary for the child as possible, which
> is hard. Letting them know that the

medical team is with them and their family will be with them. If they're having symptoms, they need to tell us. If they're scared, they need to tell us. If they have questions, they need to tell us.

These are hard conversations to have, but I think it's important for kids to know what we're thinking and know what we think is going to happen. I think it's part of them trusting us and not having us hide information from them.

In all of these fears, no matter who is afraid or of what, I think the solution is conversation. There will always be something to be afraid of in the field of pediatric cancer— fear of the diagnosis, the side effects, the test results, cancer recurrence, or death. They must be faced as a team. This is the ultimate job of the physician. By truly being present, partnering with patients and families, exploring emotions and helping to process fear, doctors are able to make cancer a little less frightening. One doctor reflects on this gift:

I find the greatest gratification in knowing that as their doctor, I was able to be there. Even though it was a really horrific situation, I was able to somehow deal with some level of suffering and make it better for them than if I hadn't been there. Because they're going through the worst time that hopefully they will ever go through in their lives. To be with them during that time is an incredible, incredible job.

Just being present with these families, answering their questions, or spending time with them helps allay their fears. This doctor thinks his time is one of the strongest supports for his patients and their families

> I think in terms of like knowing them
> well and spending a lot of time with
> them. I'm not sure you can really get
> too close. The negative to getting so
> close is that it just hurts that much more
> if they don't survive

> I think the most important thing about
> being an oncologist is spending a lot of
> time with the families. I sense a lot of
> people don't agree with that. But I think
> you need to be there in those times. I
> think, other than a physician's or a
> nurse's time, it is very difficult to give
> these people the support that they need.

For me, there is something beautiful in working with kids with cancer—shared emotions, including fears, unite doctors, patients, and families. Cancer binds us together if we recognize our own fears and discuss them with others. As healthcare providers and in general, we must process them fully by thinking and conversing about them openly. The most limiting fear is to be afraid to even have a conversation about this emotion. If one does not explore fear, the patient, the family, and the doctor will be paralyzed in an emotional isolation. That is a lonely, dark place in life as it is in cancer. Facing cancer and its fears alone from any perspective—patient, doctor, parent, or family member is insurmountable. It is better to do it together

CHAPTER 4

Faith

"Fear imprisons, faith liberates; fear paralyzes, faith empowers; fear disheartens, faith encourages; fear sickens, faith heals; fear makes useless, faith makes serviceable."

—Harry Emerson Fosdick

Faith is a powerful answer to fear. It affirms the human struggle; it supports our existence in its many forms through spirituality, morality, and commonality. Faith is able to answer the question, "Why?" for so many of us. No matter the form faith takes, its power can be stronger than that of trust. Trust flourishes when those sharing it are on equal footing and have each other's best interests at heart. Trust waxes and wanes over time, whereas faith has a more lasting trajectory; it is less influenced by outside forces and provides strength for many providers, patients, and their families. Whether it arises from organized religion or not, faith in a god, in each other, or in ourselves encourages us to persevere through the most difficult situations. It allows us to find great meaning in both life and death. In pediatric oncology, faith is often a steadfast partner in supporting the missions of patients and doctors alike. Yet, when faith does not align with medicine's ideas, it can also be a most uncompromising adversary.

My own faith is not oriented in one direction or towards one religion. It is broader and ill defined. I remember my grandfather saying, "It doesn't matter what you believe in as long as you believe in something. Believe in something larger than yourself." I am but one person moving in this wide world through time; there were many who preceded me and more will follow after. I have somehow ended up in the spot about to become a doctor preparing to treat children with cancer after my training. While my own ambition and hard work have gotten me here, so have an environment that fostered personal success and a support system of loving parents, family, friends, and mentors. Along the way, there has always been a guiding force that, in my mind, has coordinated some of this. I have depended on this faith for comfort, love, and acceptance. It has been a power that I look to in anger, happiness, frustration, gratitude, guilt, and sadness as it is my personal faith; it has always been there as an answer.

Like many tragedies, children suffering or dying from cancer can be a difficult concept to grasp in terms of fairness, reasoning, or spirituality. As one provider says:

> I mean it's terrible. It's tragic. Children are not supposed to die of cancer, but they do. That's just the way it is. [Every death] gives me something to sort of push for and to work toward.

For some providers, faith offers solace in this journey. Religion helps doctors process their patients' illnesses and cope with emotional struggles in their professional and personal lives.

One doctor explains how he deals with the stresses of his job through the lens of religion:

> I have a very supportive family... I am active in my church. My most important thing is I'm a Christian and this is not all there is. Scripture guarantees that someday there will be no more pain and suffering. That's the only thing that keeps me going, quite frankly, some days.
>
> I don't know how many of my colleagues handle this without that...

Even colleagues without the same sense of religious conviction are able to process the emotions and suffering in their own personal ways. I have met many doctors who remain centered and compassionate without religion to ground them. Though, deeply religious families can present challenges for these non-religious physicians. In reflecting on this theme, one such doctor discusses the difficulties he encounters when a family asks him to pray with them:

> I think—this is probably true in oncology practice everywhere but especially in this part of the country—a lot of people mention religion or they'll say, "My faith..." and things like that. I've never been a religious person... it's difficult for me when a family starts to become very religious or if they start to bring religion into it. It's difficult for me to support them. As an example, it's hard for me to say, "I'm praying for you,"

> because I really don't have that aspect [in
> my life]. I think a lot of doctors in
> oncology do have that religious part.
> Instead I might say "I'm thinking about
> you." For me, it's not religion, but it's
> sort of moralistic. It's like this is the right
> thing to do. Whether it's God or [a type
> of] religion, it is right to support these
> people in this setting. While I don't have
> a religious side that drives me, I think it's
> whatever my own religion is. It's my
> personal religion.

This "personal religion", whether self-defined or traditional, allows doctors to remain objective and emotionally connected while working with children with cancer and their families. It allows physicians to discuss death with children who are dying. It allows them to attend funeral after funeral of those who have died young. It allows them to remain focused in their careers while still functioning and being emotionally sound individuals in their lives outside of medicine.

Faith is a powerful force motivating many to develop and preserve a positive life outlook. It comforts patients and their families, calms their anger, presents a spiritual explanation for a cancer diagnosis or death, allows grief to fade and offers hope and direction to those who are emotionally lost. It is a guiding light. However, this same light that guides our patients and families forward can also blind them. Religious interpretations do not always align with modern medical thought. Sometimes, these differences are mere inconveniences, but occasionally they become matters of life and death.

An inconvenience is not being able to discharge a patient on time as planned. I have seen multiple Orthodox Jewish patients being held an extra day or two because their holy day is Saturday and they request not to be discharged until Sunday or later. This practice occurs even though they are medically ready for discharge. Whether insurance reimbursing thousands of dollars for these extra days is morally justified or not depends on the question of the value of religious adherence versus resource allocation. Regardless, the practice of delaying discharge in observance of faith practices is not intended to harm anyone. Yet, in a medical landscape with finite resources—beds, insurance dollars, and time of physicians and nurses—one could argue that to offer services to one person, taking the form of a non-medically necessary hospital bed in this case, is to take resources away from someone else in a direct or indirect way.

In other situations, complying with religious beliefs more plainly harms patients. This conflict of religious values with modern medicine values is evident in the healthcare of Jehovah's Witnesses. Some groups in this religion state that followers should not accept blood transfusions from others. Even in cases of massive blood loss where death is imminent without transfusions—such as traumatic injuries, childbirth with hemorrhaging, and medical conditions with non-functioning or low blood cells like leukemia and anemia—some followers will still refuse blood products or attempt to restrict them in their children. As long as an adult has made his or her wishes clear and well-documented, the medical profession has determined it is ethical to withhold blood products in adherence with these religious beliefs. However, we do not offer that same authority to children who are Jehovah's Witnesses. Doctors, ethicists, and the courts have decided that this particular religious doctrine will not be fully accommodated for children with cancer. The chemotherapy, radiation, and bone marrow transplants used to treat cancer often require many blood transfusions to keep children alive and healthy. Sometimes parameters are modified so that a child receives less blood than he or she otherwise would have normally, but only if doctors believe it can be done safely. Doctors, for the most part, graciously confront the difficulties that the blood transfusion issue presents: extra conversations, repeated nighttime consent of parents every time a child needs a blood product, and speaking with faith leaders if necessary. In this instance, the field has decided medicine's priorities trump that of religion, although we tread carefully and compassionately. Here's one quip by a doctor on the subject:

> [Religious conflicts] come up actually...
> not just with treatment but... with blood
> transfusions with Jehovah's Witnesses,
> like you [the writer] learned about in
> medical school which you thought
> you'd never deal with—except that you
> do.

Religion is pervasive and adherents are strong in their convictions. Issues and differences of opinion based on religious beliefs do arise when treating children with cancer.

I experienced this tension between faith and medicine with a fourteen-year-old patient, and I was exasperated by faith's capacity to blind the believers with devastating consequences. I only saw a brief moment of this story, but I still believe it is useful to discuss. The patient was—I am using the past tense as he has likely passed away by now—just a boy. He had been diagnosed with a type of bone tumor called an osteosarcoma, which can be treated with chemotherapy, radiation, and optional surgery with an amputation either preserving the limb or not. It is not a type of cancer with the best prognosis, but it is also not the worst. Children have a 75 to 80% chance of cure if the cancer has not metastasized, meaning that it has not spread beyond its original site. In this case, the doctors advocated for part of the limb to be amputated since the chance for survival would be significantly better even though amputations are difficult to cope with physically and emotionally. Yet, the mother refused surgery for her son because, "God was going to save [her] child," and the doctors could not dissuade her otherwise. This choice likely reduced the chance of her son surviving to about 65%.

Instead, this young boy received only chemotherapy and radiation and did not undergo surgery to amputate the limb. The cancer eventually spread to his lungs. It grew to the size of a melon on his left arm; blood vessels grew throughout the tumor. It invaded past the skin, so that tumor tissue and blood vessels were exposed and oozing on the surface of his arm. At this point, the child was in significant pain and was coming in for weekly blood transfusions, extensive wound care, and bloodwork. He was likely to die from an infection or anemia very soon. His only chance of survival was to amputate his arm. Still, his mother refused and continued saying, "God will heal you. Don't listen to them [the doctors]." The mother believed God's power to cure a child with cancer was supreme and independent of modern medicine. In the abstract, on a spiritual, intellectual, and theoretical level, these questions are stimulating. But I believe in this situation, her beliefs were non-pragmatic and damaging. This mother's conviction was strong and I respect her faith, but I find it difficult to respect her decision.

I was angry at the mother. I don't know for certain if the outcome would have been better if she'd allowed the amputation to proceed, but her insistence and blind faith infuriated me. Denial is a strong beast, but faith dwarfed denial's power in this situation. She did not agree with her son using a wheelchair when he was weak; she instead kept insisting that, "God was going to save him." The physical and emotional pain it must have caused her son is unimaginable. Furthermore, I wonder about the doctors and the rest of the treatment team: the nurses, social workers, and support staff. How had no one gotten through to this woman and aligned her faith with the goals of medicine while respecting both? I'm sure they tried, but how could they not have succeeded for the sake of her son, their patient? I desperately wished that they could have broken her faith at least a little.

Multiple emotions intersect in this boy's story for me and cloud complete understanding. This mother loved her son and didn't want him to die. She truly believed her view and acted in accordance with complete trust and faith in her God. The choices she made ran counter to the ones I or modern medicine support. Her rationale continues to battle me, and the difference of opinions is vast. I am left with such awe at the power of her faith. I have profound empathy for the pain and sorrow she must have suffered. I cannot imagine her experience and her decision to leave her son in the hands of God, refusing the interventions of modern medicine, and undoubtedly enduring many blatant or veiled dismissive comments from providers. She was his mother. She had fourteen years with her son. She watched him grow, raised him, and was there through all of his life experiences: first word, first steps, first day of school, and the first day he learned of his cancer. How strong a conviction is necessary to refuse treatment in this way? How deep is her faith to put trust for her son's cure in God over medicine? Did God disappoint her? Would her faith change after her son passed away?

Faith is never simple. It exists in more permutations than any other human idea because faith is inherently individual and is primarily between a person and a divine being or beings. A person's relationship with faith is unique and deeply personal. This is the reason why faith, as it relates to pediatric oncology, is arguably the hardest to conceptualize. It, like other emotions or ideas, is not based on scientific reason, but rather on a "feeling". People spend their whole lives defining their own set of values and beliefs. Thus, it is impossible for a clinician to fully understand a patient's faith and its implications on medical care during an encounter or illness experience.

Overall however, faith is mostly a positive force. Doctors and families are able to harness its power to motivate patients, reassure them, and give them perspective in their struggles. It is one of the most helpful mechanisms in illness and at the end of life. One doctor reflects on the role of faith in her conversations with a young girl:

> Probably the youngest child that I have talked directly with about dying was seven years old. This was a child, not someone who had cancer, but a young girl who had a degenerative neurologic disease, end-stage kidney disease, and was on a respirator. I talked with her about the fact that the respirator was going to be removed and that we hoped

she would be able to breathe on her
own, but we knew that that was going to
be very hard.

And that maybe even though she tried
hard she wouldn't be able to do that. If
she couldn't do that it meant that she
would die and go to Heaven. There
would be people waiting for her there,
like her grandmother. She was Catholic,
and I knew that she believed in the
afterlife. I knew that her grandmother
had died the year before and I said,
"Your grandmother will be there, and
she'll be waiting for you. You and your
grandmother will be able to do some of
the things that you've missed doing with
her."

That was very comforting to this child;
to just have the sense that she was going
to a place where there would be
someone who would know her and she
wouldn't be all alone.

In this conversation is everything that faith can be. It
calls forth fellowship, meaning, and love into a world where
there is too little of all three. Faith in humanity, each other,
our gods, or within our personal religion, is a bright light in
medicine. It allows doctors to wake up in the morning with
purpose and perspective. It allows parents and families to
emotionally and spiritually cope when their loved ones have
cancer. Finally, it allows patients, children of all ages, to
find support and meaning in their cancer, to find significance

in their lives and even in their deaths. Faith empowers; it is truly a beautiful gift.

CHAPTER 5

Sadness
Patients

"You who have not lost do not yet know how infinite pain is."

Elizabeth Hall Hunter, *From the cross*, in Life with Sam

Sadness is perhaps the most transferable of emotions. It jumps from one individual to another with such ease and stealth as compared to other emotions. When observing a happy, carefree toddler in the park, one feels a ripple of happiness, maybe enough to smile. But when looking even at a photograph of a grieving mother, we become absorbed in sadness. For many, being in the presence of someone crying makes the witness feel similar intense grief. Whether we read sad stories, listen to accounts, watch movies, or experience our own personal sadness, this emotion makes a stronghold in our core. We are consumed with emotion. In that moment it takes from us a sliver of our past happiness, connection, hope, love, or humanity. Its effect is to leave us feeling alone and hollow with a changed sense of self and order in the world. Sadness replaces our being with emptiness piece by piece. That is why it is so painful. Its prerogative is to longitudinally erode our emotional identity into one solely defined by sadness.

The theme of sadness occurs throughout medicine; it accompanies grave illnesses and tragic outcomes. It occupies patients and their families. It also, to a varying degree, inflicts its emotional damage on providers—doctors, nurses, and support staff—who work in the field. To witness and share suffering of patients is deep and difficult, but it is also gratifying. It is a feeling of privilege to partner with patients in their illnesses, health, triumphs, and even their deaths. Doctors have an almost carte blanche access to their patients' worlds and bodies. This remarkable intimacy is needed to best provide treatment, which includes the physical care of the patient's body and the emotional care of the person. Perhaps the greatest offering by a patient or family is to openly invite a provider to share in sadness. For these children and families to display their vulnerability, grief, and pain in front of providers who are largely strangers is a meaningful demonstration of the trust and emotional need in medicine. These poignant moments are profound and moving.

In pediatric oncology, there are certainly tones of sadness. Yet, these tones mix with many other emotional chords. In hearing the initial diagnosis, sadness may blend with shock. In treatment proving unable to cure the disease, sadness may swell with anger or denial. Even in the case of survival or cure, sadness may persist veiled in regret for lost opportunities. And in death, sadness may seem insurmountable in its overwhelming loneliness and tragedy. Its forms are varied, and its reach is far. From sadness' epicenter around a child with cancer, its influence extends towards families, communities, and providers. In each domain, its impact is strong and its lessons are lasting. Despite the pain and suffering, there is growth. That is one of the saving grace of sadness within pediatric oncology. As one doctor said:

> Every child and every family really leaves something to you. The beauty of the job is not only the science, but it is what you are gaining as a person, what these families and those kids give you... when you recall their stories. In taking care of each kid and each family, they have given you something that will help you later either with your personal or professional life.

What follows is a selection of patient and family stories that have been meaningful to me in their sadness. Some are from first hand experience and others were told to me about patients by the oncologists I interviewed. All are beautiful in their emotional gravity and raw truth. I struggled in writing this chapter. To share the stories seems a double edged sword. They are not my stories. I wonder if I have broken a covenant of trust that is implied when patients invite us to share in their sadness. I am editing their stories in the telling, and I wonder if the reduction of a life experience to a brief narrative can adequately capture the complexity of emotions and convey it authentically. These patients and their illnesses are more than merely stories of sadness. Even in the devastation there is hope, love, and even happiness.

To assign levels of sadness in children with cancer is almost preposterous. Yet, I think it is something we subconsciously do and don't often discuss. Some situations evoke more vivid feelings than others. In my own experience, the children that affected me most were those that suffered alone. Cancer inflicts much emotional anguish, but in a united, loving family, this can be tempered. But if cancer is joined with isolation, the descent into worsening sadness seems inevitable.

I remember a very young patient, a six-month-old baby girl with Down syndrome and leukemia. I would play with her and swell with joy as she smiled and looked into my eyes. Yet, I also felt a deep pang of anger and sadness for what I considered the cruelty of fate. She was born with Down syndrome, a genetic disorder associated with characteristic physical and facial features as well as intellectual disabilities. In an unfair twist of genetics, those with Down syndrome also have an increased risk of cancer, specifically leukemia. She had both. Her family had abandoned her after she became sick. They hadn't come to visit her in weeks and her mother had avoided all contact by providers. To look at this young baby without a care in the world, cooing with attention when the nurses and I played with her broke my heart. We called her "Bella", which means beauty. Her darling demeanor was a stark contrast to her tragic family environment. Her cancer was very likely to be cured, and she would probably live a long and healthy life. But whenever I think about her, my thoughts descend towards misery because I remember that her family deserted her. This is one of cancer's most disastrous although rare side effects: isolation to the extreme of abandonment. She was not the only child I saw who was abandoned after their illness was diagnosed. It hurts to imagine explaining to a child that she was abandoned because she had cancer. It pains me to a level of sadness that I cannot describe. To me, it seems that the universe follows its own rules when distributing sadness and does not entertain the notion of fairness. Some seem fated to suffer more than others, leaving those of us spared to watch from the sidelines, intervening when compelled.

Sadness seems to be an emotion without limits insatiable. It consorts with other emotions in dangerous combinations. When it does so it is a force to be reckoned with. Loneliness multiplies the effects of sadness and infuses it with power. For if one is alone, there is no support in the fight against sadness. Cancer is an alienating disease especially in the pediatric population. Children are taken out of school for months at a time for treatment, they often lose their hair, and their worlds become filled with medical staff and hospitals. In thinking about one twelve-year-old boy, there was a unique version of the sadness in his story of being called "cancer boy" at school. To have the self-awareness to realize you are different is one thing, but to be reminded of it through bullying and social isolation is quite another. Even in children who can't clearly vocalize their sadness, we know the feeling is present. This emotional awareness was demonstrated by a charming three-year-old boy who had neuroblastoma, a solid tumor of the nervous system. During one of our discussions with his parents about treatment and discharge, he interrupted by jumping up and standing in his hospital crib. He started whimpering, his eyes filled with tears as he looked up at all of us, and in the softest, high-pitched little boy voice, he simply said, "I'm sad." We were all stunned by the truth he told about himself. He knew what it meant to be sad, and he felt the urge to share it with us in his own way. He wanted to be heard.

The feelings evoked in these moments never fade. Sadness seems to lodge itself in memories that last forever. When triggered, the feeling recollected may appear with less intensity and more perspective than originally felt. Yet, the feelings evoked for the story-teller and the audience can be reawakened through these stories. Doctors sometimes forget patients, but they tend to remember even the smallest details of those they felt were their saddest patients. One doctor is reminded of a previous patient whenever she sees a school bus:

> His name was Johnny, he was five, and he had a brain tumor. He was supposed to go to kindergarten next year and his sister was supposed to go into the second grade. So, she had been riding the school bus, and this was the thing that he was most excited about for kindergarten. He was excited to ride the school bus. So, he said to his mother in late August before he died, "When I'm an angel in Heaven, will I be able to ride the school bus?" And she said, "Yes."
>
> He's a little boy that I think of whenever I see a school bus—an angel riding in a school bus.

Families often feel sad and overwhelmed simultaneously. They are emotional partners that feed into each other and are synergistic in their potential to prevent people from seeking and accepting help. One overwhelmed mother illustrates this concept best. Her daughter had AML, a type of leukemia, and all those around her, including the doctors, had seen that the mother was falling apart. She increasingly became consumed by her sadness, and that bred anger and depression. She refused to see a psychiatrist or accept any mental health counseling to work with her feelings. Her responses to well intentioned inquiries became increasingly defensive and eventually turned into, "Stop asking how I am." She retreated more and more from discussions involving emotion. Her sadness had succeeded in isolating her.

Sadness is not a simple emotion. It contains a multitude of dimensions. As shown above, sadness flourishes in negativity; it grows in fear and anger. But sadness can also paradoxically inspire beauty, meaning, and love.

> Recently, we had a patient who passed away. He was eleven years old. He had AML [a type of leukemia] and multiple relapses after transplant. He had started on Phase I and Phase II therapy; after a month of it, he started to have symptoms again and came in.
>
> His mom found he'd been flushing his medications and they sat down with him... and he said, "I'm tired." He completely understood what it meant to be flushing his medications. He knew he wasn't going to survive. He's like, "I can't do this anymore."
>
> That would be devastating for parents, [especially] if they aren't to that point yet... suddenly realizing their child is at that point is hard to imagine. I could not contemplate being in that situation. I would hope I would reach that [decision] at the same time as my child. These were

parents who very much wanted to keep pushing and they were pushing.

Their child, sort of behind their back, was like, "I'm not doing this." At a certain point you can't make the child do something that they don't want to do. While the parents have the legal right to say, yes, we're going to keep treating, he's going to flush his medications.

I can't imagine a family would push him. It's not like they're going to put down a nasogastric tube [a tube down his nose into his stomach for administering food or medications]; I hope they wouldn't. I think at that point it [transitions] into supportive care and trying to help the family come to grips. They did fairly quickly. It was devastating when they first realized [he was flushing his pills]. But by the time they'd gotten here to the hospital, after learning this, they'd already... started to realize that this was [the end].

When it becomes clear that a child is going to die of cancer and everyone knows it, sadness is definitely present. Yet, it can be managed with deliberate actions from all those involved: patients, families, and doctors who have gone through the process hundreds of times. While it's heart-wrenching to think about, families have certain choices in experiencing their sadness if they understand they are at the end. One family demonstrated this thoughtful acceptance at the end of a young man's life. They chose to still treat with chemotherapy even though it was unlikely to prolong his life, but they scheduled it around other priorities. This approach helped to diminish their sadness. He was a seventeen year old young man with recurrent rhabdomyosarcoma, a type of soft tissue tumor. He had been through the gamut of treatment options and nothing had worked. He was left frustrated as the investigational therapy turned his hair a stark white color. He was disgusted as the tumor had grown into his mouth and bits of the tumor would flake off into his mouth. As he said, "it is what it is." The whole family had come to the clinic for his outpatient appointment and the room was palpably tense. They were there to talk about end of life planning even though they really didn't want to. They were going on "one last" family vacation to a beach and wanted to make sure plans were in place if he got sick on the vacation; so there they were. The sadness saturated that clinic room. The conversation was one of lasts, last breaths, vacations, prescriptions, and memories. But in that sadness of lasts, were threads of hope and happiness. If he lived through this family vacation, the plan was to restart another cycle of chemotherapy. The boy felt comforted, "as long as we're doing something." The mom felt her maternal instinct to protect and care for her son was fulfilled, "I feel good because we're doing something." The boy would certainly not survive many more months, but this plan to restart chemotherapy was something they needed. They needed this future goal to keep going in the moment.

Everyone experiences sadness differently. In pediatric oncology, the variety is strikingly demonstrated through the multitude of unique end of life journeys. In the last couple months of a child's life, the variance of feelings and choices is so personal. One doctor reflects on helping his patients and families make the best choices for them at the end:

> In those situations, I've learned that it's not my job to tell them what to do. It's my job to facilitate what they want. If they want to stop, that's fine with me, and I will work on getting hospice and palliative care set up. If they want to [enroll in] every phase I trial and see every developmental oncologist and developmental therapeutic program, then I will do my best to make that happen too—within what is safe and reasonable. At the end of the day, if you know the patient is going to die, especially when it's a child, there are going to be people who remain.
>
> They have to be able to live with themselves and the decisions that they have made. If it's the kind of family where they're not going to be able to feel like they did everything for their child if we didn't try—even though it's futile and maybe it's putting them through unnecessary things—if everybody is on board, then you have to do that. It's not like you [the doctor] are the one driving the boat anymore. You become the director, but not the captain. You help and you facilitate, but you are not the one actually making the decisions...

How does a family want to live out that
time?

To decide as a family how to spend a child's last days
or weeks… to watch a child drift towards death unaware
because parents think she is too young to know… to listen to
a mother tell you "I have many children" because her only
child is about to die of cancer… to watch a child hooked up
to an oxygen mask struggling to breathe and screaming, "I'm
drowning! I'm drowning!" because leukemia has
compromised his lungs… to witness an adolescent give away
her computer because she, "won't need it anymore"… to
answer a child's question, "Am I going to die?"… to see
cancer hurt children and to witness the anguish, unfairness,
and cruelty of it all. These are the feelings of sadness in
pediatric oncology. Sadness is unlike any other emotion in
that it is a portal that we can revisit forever. When we are
touched by sadness, it becomes a fixed memory of feeling,
time, and place. We can reaccess it and all of its details at a
moment's notice. Listening to doctors across the country
reflect on their patients and the theme of sadness, I
witnessed them transported to other places when they
relayed these stories. They seemed to relive each moment
and each patient's journey in front of me.

The stories always had the same effect on me. They
made the room feel cold, slowed time, blurred the
environment in a haze, and reinforced that I had never really
known this level of sadness. All of the stories dwarfed and
shamed my personal life experiences of sadness. I think that
is one of the powerful lessons in pediatric oncology. In
exploring others' circumstances, you develop more
understanding of your own emotions and you gain
perspective on your own sadness. Each time that cloud of

sadness lifts, we are left with a sense of stillness and appreciation for the larger meaning in these stories and experiences. Its departure requires perspective and support from ourselves and others. Sadness, like any other emotion, demands to be felt. I ask you to feel it, talk about it, and explore it.

CHAPTER 6

Shock

"There is a feeling of disbelief that comes over you, that takes over and you kind of go through the motions. You do what you're supposed to do, but in fact you're not there at all."

Frederick Barthelme, *Elroy Nights*

Shock is the absence of emotion. It enters with no warning and blindsides with rapidity and completeness. This feeling catapults its targets into a void from which they are unable to recognize their own position. Shock is so overwhelming that it precludes other emotions from being felt concurrently. If a person is in shock, he is unable to process further information much less other feelings. Shock waits in the background. It creeps throughout life and medicine and prepares to pounce. It presents itself to doctors in an unexpected outcome, a scientific breakthrough, or a rare, dreaded side effect of a drug. It disrupts the lives of patients in an untimely diagnosis or surprise in either a positive or negative way, and it thrusts families into a predicament; they become unable to support each other, stunned motionless in a blank stare at the precise moment when they require the most support. This is an emotion that enters pediatric oncology quickly and exits almost automatically with the same speed. It isn't able to sustain any true longevity. That is the saving grace of shock. It is brutal, but short-lived.

As a medical student, you learn how to manage your feelings and response to situations. There are many lessons about emotions implicit and explicit in the curriculum. Perhaps one of the most direct is that shock is an emotion never to be displayed by a clinician. A shocked doctor is perceived by patients to be casting judgment; and "providers should never judge their patients". In my years as a medical student, I've learned to minimize my inner feelings of shock and completely extinguish my external display of this emotion. It is a peculiar skill, but one which I see useful for a doctor to have. To not appear shocked when your patient and her mother are telling you blatant lies about actions you have personally witnessed, to listen to ridiculous verbal arguments, and to work with some truly outrageous patients without exuding any reaction to their absurdities requires much self-control. This is especially true when gathering a history. You really have to be in medicine to understand how shocking patients' behavior can be or relate to some of the things they are capable of saying. Oftentimes I am extremely shocked, even if I never show it.

Experienced doctors work through their shock efficiently and completely. Perhaps repeated similar insults build up a shock-tolerance of sorts in pediatric oncology. Looking at blood under the microscope and confirming cancer does not retain its same level of shock after the first couple times. Screaming, squirming children are less of a challenge after one performs many exams and procedures on similar children. In a way, routine is the result of repeated shock no matter the absurdity of the inciting factors. Yet, even with all the tolerance built up, situations still shock doctors. The aftermath of these situations is most often a contemplative reevaluation. This may lead to a redirection of treatment course or an analysis of how shock crept into the situation. Doctors aim to be confident and composed. Shock disrupts their routines, and therefore serves little purpose in medicine. It should be prevented when possible. Repetition and patterns both insulate from shock and create it when cases don't fit the mold. Doctors become comfortable with expected outcomes; they see common as common. When rare outcomes happen, they can be shock, especially in young doctors who haven't seen all the exceptions occur. For example, a child with standard risk acute lymphoblastic leukemia (ALL), a type of blood cancer, has a greater than 90% chance of being cured. That is the typical pattern, and it becomes almost expected that these children will be cured. A physician recounts a patient who was the exception:

> He was about four when he was diagnosed. He had standard-risk leukemia. So, at the very end of therapy, I thought, "Okay, we're done. Go out and play baseball!" But, we did his end of therapy bone marrow and he had 50% blasts [markers of cancer in the blood], which is crazy. I remember looking… and we were in pathology rounds, and after double checking, he had blasts in there. I [remember thinking], "No way. There's no way. This can't possibly be."

To see a child's end of therapy test reveal that the treatment failed to work when in the vast majority of cases it is "supposed" to work upsets the status quo of expectations. It humbles and jolts doctors into a whirlwind of emotions. Cancer has an incessant need to remind us that it does not play by the rules and is not fair. Its capacity to shock is great for doctors, families, and patients. As Kristine Wyllys in her book, *Losing Streak,* says:

> Cancer, he'd said near the end, is the great equalizer. It doesn't care who you are or what kind of salary you make. It doesn't give one damn if you are a good person or a bad one. It is the ultimate villain because it's not capable of mercy. It only knows how to destroy and that's exactly what it does. Destroys everything.

Doctors are shocked by more than just unexpected treatment or disease outcomes. Sometimes a family's decision to go against medical recommendations causes immense incredulity akin to shock. Guided by compassion and expertise, doctors almost always have a preferred direction for those gray areas in medicine. This occurs in pediatric oncology when doctors want to be more aggressive in attempting cure and survival than families and patients want to be. Most of the time, everyone wants to be aggressive in seeking a cure. Therefore, when patients or families do not want to treat early in the course, it can be very shocking. Many advocate for patient autonomy, and this is noble and true in many situations. Yet, patient autonomy is challenging for the doctors if they perceive the families' choice as misguided. A physician relayed to me a situation involving a seventeen-year-old boy who had osteosarcoma, a type of bone tumor, in his leg. The family had chosen to forego surgery to remove the tumor because it would require a metal rod to be placed in his femur, and they believed this was "unnatural". Yet, the family and boy agreed to treat with chemotherapy alone. When surgery is combined with chemotherapy, the chance of cure is around 70%. When chemotherapy is used alone, the cure rate is worse, at about 55 to 60%. Doctors were shocked to learn of this decision and the underlying thought process. In their opinion, the surgery wasn't even an amputation. It was only a metal rod, and the surgery wasn't anymore "unnatural" than chemotherapy. Accepting toxic chemicals, but not a metal rod; this situation was shocking to them:

> The family came to us and said, "We're not comfortable with surgery," because the surgery consisted of taking off part of his bone and putting in a metal rod. "We're not comfortable with having a piece of metal in his leg. That's not appropriate to us. That seems very unnatural." It would've been in his proximal femur. That took everyone by surprise, [them] saying that.

> [The patient] had multiple meetings with his primary oncologist, his radiation oncologist, and the orthopedic doctor. There were probably at least three big meetings about this... the family stood strong and kept saying, "We understand there are risks. We don't want the metal rod." This was so unusual. I mean, you just don't hear people say that.

> It's really hard. I think our obligation is to involve other physicians and ethicists

to try to push for the best option for the child. In this case, they didn't refuse all therapy, they just refused one portion. As best as we can guess, this is around a 10 to 15% difference in survival… Most people felt like a 10 to 15% difference was not enough to try to go to the courts and take custody of care, especially complicated by the fact that he was seventeen years. He was just about eighteen…

I don't think that happens much. That case is really rare. It's rare that a family would, especially after understanding and having major family meetings and everything, would do something that clearly has a worse outcome.

Pediatric oncologists balance length of life and quality as paramount in their goals of treatment. When parents or children make choices counterintuitive to both those pursuits, it can be quite shocking. In this emotion's wake, doctors must decide whether to attempt to persuade their patients or to follow their "ill-perceived" decisions. On this level of patient autonomy, one doctor seemed to think his families received too much.

I think autonomy is "everything" nowadays. I think we probably as a society give families too much autonomy, that's my own view. There's no way a family could understand all the details of these regimens. I think families

wind up deciding based on what their
doctor thinks and lifestyle: how hard will
the child take it, that kind of thing.

Shock happens especially when patients and families
hear a diagnosis of cancer for the first time. In the days or
weeks leading up to a diagnosis, parents may have noticed or
begun to suspect something is seriously wrong with their
child. Their pediatrician may have even mentioned the
possibility of cancer or conducted preliminary tests to
determine its likelihood. In some cases, the emergency room
physician confirms the diagnosis before consulting an
oncologist. But, often the pediatric oncologist is the one to
share this information and clearly articulate to the parents
and child that the diagnosis is cancer. This is a substantial
responsibility and one which always conjures shock in the
family, no matter the preceding course. An oncologist
reflects on this initial shock:

> The person to whom you're going to
> give the news has been expecting it, but
> hoping and praying that you're not going
> to give them that news. So, when it does
> come, it's not exactly a shock, it's putting
> the final reality to a fear they have had.
> It's extremely important that you realize
> that. Because of the level of shock,
> they're going to remember little of what
> you tell them; it's going to be important
> to say things many times over. You'll
> have to repeat several times during the
> course of that initial interview in giving
> them the diagnosis.

Remember when they come back a day, an hour, or a week later, and say, "But, you never told me." Realize that although you may have told them, it was too much for them to understand and take in [completely]. There's a level of denial that people have that helps them to get the news in chunks rather than all at once. Part of that denial is not to hear [information].

People will come back and say, "But, you never told me. I didn't realize it was this bad. You didn't tell me what I was supposed to do." That's a common thing that is sometimes frustrating...

It's important that they have an opportunity to ask questions, but don't be surprised if they don't have any at that time. Some of the questions are too scary to ask or contemplate, so they don't ask a question. They may ask it later... When you're going to have the family meeting, it's really important to have several members of the family present if possible. [Based] on their relationship, people are going to be hit by the news in different ways.

For example, if there's an aunt or uncle there as opposed to just the parents, they have the advantage of being one step removed. In most cases, it's easier for them to hear the news, be able to ask questions, and interpret back.

This theme of shock disrupting information processing occurs in parents who have just received the news. It is so prevalent that one oncologist has this piece built into her script when she shares a new cancer diagnosis:

> In my day one talk, I always say, "You will remember 3% of what we talk about today. That's it. Everybody does that. Don't worry about it. We can have this conversation one hundred more times." I do think that sometimes all they hear is cancer. Other times they refuse to hear the word cancer.

The most shocking time for families and patients in their entire cancer journeys is likely to be when they hear that initial diagnosis. But, as alluded to above, they often suspect something serious before the diagnosis is confirmed. As this oncologist says:

> Most families know first of all. Often, they know something is really wrong. Sometimes, it's a relief to have an answer, although not really a relief to have an answer.

Doctors have the advantage of planning when approaching this situation. Their knowledge of its occurrence and content allows them to plan the conversation ahead of time. Thus, the doctor is able to manage shock and perhaps preempt it with careful handling while delivering the news to the child and family.

Families and patients tend to be shocked even more by abrupt changes in treatment plans or diagnostic information than by the initial diagnosis. In medicine, as in life, nothing always goes as planned. In fact, while shock from hearing the initial diagnosis tends to withdraw to calm and understanding; shock that is provoked by a deviation from what was originally thought or planned for can leave anger and mistrust in its wake. This is a dangerous situation in medicine. Medicine is a field of learning through apprenticeship, thus providers are of varying experience and there is a steep learning curve. These trainee levels include medical students, first-year doctors called interns, junior doctors called residents, more senior though still training doctors called fellows, and the most senior doctors who supervise, called attendings. Clinical care is provided by all those above with many checks and balances to ensure high quality, effective care. Junior members of the team attempt to convey accurate information appropriate to their training level and avoid missteps. But mistakes do still happen.

One of those mistakes is to misinform patients by telling them incorrect information or treatment plans. Sometimes all it takes is a swift correction of the misinformation, but sometimes it isn't so easy. Below is a scenario of an eleven-year-old girl who came in to an outpatient oncology clinic with seborrheic dermatitis, a skin condition, and rheumatoid arthritis. She has been having fevers, joint pain, and swollen lymph nodes for weeks which concerned her primary care provider as signs of cancer. So, he referred her to the oncology clinic for further evaluation.

The fellow saw the patient first alone. Here is a snapshot of the end of the encounter:

> Girl: "Why did I have to come all the way here?"
>
> Fellow: "You are here to find out from us that you don't have cancer."
>
> Mom: "Woohoo, you don't have cancer!"
>
> Girl: "Told you so!" *followed by high-fiving her mom.*
>
> Mom: "What do we do from here?"
>
> Fellow: *As leaving the room,* "Go see a rheumatologist and dermatologist."

Once the fellow left the room, she consulted with the senior oncologist, the attending. He disagreed, felt it was possible that this was cancer, and wanted to perform further tests. While swollen lymph nodes, fevers, and joint pain could be symptoms of her already known health conditions, they could also be signs of leukemia happening in concert with her other diagnoses. So, they both delivered this update with a drastic change of information: this could still be cancer and they needed a chest x-ray, lab tests, and to look at a blood smear with a microscope to figure it out. This came as quite the shock considering the mom and daughter had just been elatedly high-fiving moments before.

This is a basic form of shock and perhaps the most damaging. It occurs when patients are told one thing and another happens. It is one of the reasons that doctors hedge their bets or warn of rare side effects. Causing patients to worry by preparing them for a scenario which is unlikely to happen is overall less emotionally harmful than to not tell a patient and the shocking outcome somehow occurs. In pediatric oncology, the classic example that I've seen is doctors telling a patient she won't lose her hair because the chosen type of chemotherapy tends to not cause hair loss. Turns out, in the rare but possible exception that the patient's body reacts by losing her hair, families are furious and the shock is quite extreme. It is much more emotionally painful than if they had been prepared for the slight possibility of hair loss and it doesn't occur.

Doctors create shock if they do not properly diagnose a patient's condition. This is a shock to be avoided in medicine because when it leaves patients and their families, it does not heal with the usual remedy of time. It leaves an emotional void which is often permanently filled with maladaptive negative emotions. This is often anger, depression, or mistrust. It is shock in its most devilish form, and it occurs when doctors act in error:

> He was a two-year-old boy who presented to the hospital with an Ewings-like sarcoma (a type of soft tissue solid cancer). His mom took him to the pediatrician multiple times for over a year because he had a bump on his left hand which wasn't going away. The pediatrician had been saying it's a "cyst" all along and, "just to watch it."

Finally, after the lump continued to grow, the pediatrician finally recommended a biopsy and follow-up with an oncologist near the one year mark of having the bump. All this time, the cancer had been growing. Since the biopsy—which confirmed cancer, "it began to grow really fast" according to the mom and grew to the size of a large gumball on his tiny hand. By the time he came to the hospital, it was widely metastatic, meaning it had spread from the original location on his hand to his armpit, blood vessels, bones, and skull. The cancer was all over his body. What started as a small "knot" on his left hand was now likely to kill him. His complaints included pain, limited movement of his hand as he couldn't wiggle his fingers, weight loss, and another new bump in his left armpit, which his mom found. All of these signs and symptoms point to cancer. The pediatric oncologist who saw this case with me lamented that although they would give him chemotherapy and he would respond well, his cancer would recur within a year because it had spread so far before treatment was initiated.

To get cancer is tragic. To get cancer in this way is something more excruciating than tragic. As I think about this story, ripples of shock run through me almost immediately and leave me with regret when they recede. I am left letdown by the primary care doctor and angry that our system didn't treat this child earlier. I can only imagine the bottomless pain and emotions the family must be feeling to this day. The child has most likely passed away by now leaving in his wake lasting shock and regret. Maybe this is the rare example in which the shock never completely passes, no matter the time or counseling.

At first thought, it seems the most shocking conversation to have would be that you or child is going to die. Some might think it would be such a surprise to hear that a child's cancer has become incurable. Yet, it really does not seem to be the case; this conversation almost never provokes much shock. It is perhaps because this realization happens in progressive micro-shocks. One day the treatment doesn't seem to working as well. The next visit the doctor returns with mixed results. Weeks later the child is back in the hospital with a new complication. It seems that shock isn't able to enter the consciousness as much because the understanding of the changing prognosis and impending death occurs slowly over a long time course. Shock has no stamina; it must exert its influence in one shot and not over many weeks or months. One doctor talks about her strategy to inform families that a child's cancer has become incurable. She has this conversation gradually over weeks or months as the situation allows:

> It is rare that I have been in a situation where I had to switch the conversation completely, 180 degrees, from saying that this is something that we hope to cure versus this is incurable. This happens little by little even if [the doctor] already knows that we are heading to an

incurable disease. I usually go little by little because then they can adjust. At the end, [the parents and child] need to have thought about the possibility before you actually tell them.

Once they see that things have not worked, are not working as expected, and every time you do an intervention, the physician is coming back with a mixed result. "Well, it didn't work as well." "Well, it didn't work." I think in their minds, it starts building. They think that they are losing ground... Probably in their minds, they are actually unsure. They think about the possibility that the outcome will not be good and that they may eventually lose that child. Every family has this thought once a diagnosis of cancer is made.

I don't think any of them hears a diagnosis of cancer and thinks, "Okay this will be hard, but she will be cured 100%." Even if they say that, I think they know that it is not the case.

So, the moment when you say this is incurable is unlikely to come as a complete shock. Over the course, we have given them clues that this may be difficult. The moment you actually tell them, it is what they never wanted to hear, but what has been in their minds already.

Her strategy of slowly informing the families is aimed to minimize shock. In many ways, grief will be the same because the disease course wouldn't differ. It is just as sad no matter how you learn the facts. Doctors aim to tell their patients and families bad news with compassion and clarity. Sometimes though, it seems they are so afraid to shock that they hide behind vague language to dampen the shock-inducing factor. This approach confuses patients and families. It is something to consider avoiding. In pediatric oncology, doctors sometimes still avoid directly saying, "You are going to die." As this doctor states:

> You usually don't need to use those words. Occasionally when denial is the battle and they won't see reality then yes, I have to use very direct words. What I've found is the more direct you are in the short run, there's usually more pain and angst. But in the long run, it usually is much easier on the family and everybody else.

> Most of the time—there are studies documenting this—parents notice changes and figure it out. When you say, "I don't have any more therapy, all we can do at this point is hope we can find something to slow things down or treat symptoms," you might [otherwise just] say, "I have nothing that can cure him." I will use those words. That's probably a

better way to say it than, "You are going
to die."

To be honest, I'm not sure what the best words to use are.
Ambiguity in language can sometimes be employed to avoid
shocking people. Ambiguous language can veil criticism and
soften harsh brutal honesty. It can be a sugarcoating of the
true meaning of a statement. This reading between the lines
is common in medicine. It's a strategy that is used because
doctors feel it allows them to have more compassionate
conversations and to give the news softer. It feels brutal to
say, "You are going to die." But in that shocking declaration,
there is no confusion. And perhaps confusion is worse than
shock in some cases. People need to hear the truth. It needs
to be said with compassion and clarity, as noted above, but
hard topics do not need to be danced around. This can be
even more harmful.

Shock is painful to endure and witness. Victims
become paralyzed and unable to process information; those
nearby become uncomfortable in trying to support such a
helpless individual. They must wait until its control recedes,
access the damage, and then formulate a plan in its wake.
Shock occurs throughout medicine and has played a role in
shaping the art of clinical care. Doctors have found different
ways to address the emotion of shock. Most suppress it in
themselves or at least its outward manifestations. Many
attempt to lessen its blow by preparing patients gradually and
for all possible outcomes. One wonders if shock should be
avoided so completely. How hard must we work to avoid it,
and what benefits does that provide to patients and
providers? Perhaps shock should not be feared but
embraced.

CHAPTER 7

Understanding
How Doctors Break the News

"I am the sky and nothing can stick to me. The sky is open and vast and stays unchanged no matter what; it is always the sky. A storm can roll through it, an airplane can roar through, and it is always the sky."

—Geralyn Lucas, *Why I Wore Lipstick: To My Mastectomy*

Hearing a pediatric cancer diagnosis is a crushing blow. Regardless of the conversational dance or compassionate manner a doctor employs, this diagnostic sledgehammer drastically shakes a family's emotional core. In doing so, cancer changes people; it becomes part of their existence and reshapes their identity. That day, that moment, when cancer is introduced into a person's life is analogous to a rebirth, albeit tragic, for the patient and family. It is the beginning of a cruel stage production where the antagonist, Cancer, always plays the same malicious role.

Despite the changes in cast and minor script alterations, the set remains the same. It's often a blue and white hospital room, abuzz with ticking machines and incessant beeps. The opening scene tends to feel the same; it is overflowing with confusion, helplessness, anxiety, shock, sadness, and glimpses of determination. Each time a doctor utters those words, "You have cancer," it sounds like it is leaving his lips for the first time. Just before that moment, the surrounding environment for the participants fades into the background and uncertainty hangs poised above. The physician's words seem to shift gravity, to have such clarity, and with each pronunciation, a ringing lasting quality. The patient and family crumble, but the hospital walls and nearby staff have heard those words of new cancer innumerable times; they barely shudder standing stoically as families melt into their emotions and begin the transition to a new existence—one with cancer playing a predominate, central role. It is one of the most striking scenes that can occur in this play of life and is unforgettable for these patients and families. They will forget many details of that initial day, driven to the far recesses of their minds, but that feeling and that scene will stick with them forever.

In many ways, sharing a cancer diagnosis is one of the most artful demonstrations of providing family-centered healthcare. Ushering a patient into this new life is representative of medicine in its truest, most beautiful form. Communication, knowledge, and compassion intersect as the necessary components for success in this arena. It takes a skilled doctor to do it well. Telling a diagnosis of cancer is nuanced and requires many elements.

Every oncologist has different components in his or her script, but almost all include an introduction to the diagnosis, a discussion of the prognosis tailored to the capacity to understand this information, and a plan for treatment options. They often start with asking the parents and patient of their initial understanding of what is going on.

One doctor starts by asking:

> "What do you understand? What do you understand as to why you were sent to the hospital?" Some of them think it was because they had an abnormal blood test, but it's no big deal. Some of them have been told by a doctor that their child has leukemia.
>
> Obviously you're going to approach those differently. Some parents were told their child has leukemia and then the entire way here in the car they were on the web reading, and so they come here with a fairly good understanding.

Similarly, another doctor says:

> In the first day, I think it's most important to recognize that it's not just the patient that you're speaking to, it's not just the parents that you're speaking to, it's really the patient and the parents. It's very important to gauge their level of understanding.

This provides a starting point to make sure everyone is on the same page. It is a common strategy:

> So the way I usually start those conversations is by asking, "What is it that you understand so far?" because people pick up all kinds of information

from all kinds of sources, some of it medical, some of it from the person who brings the lunch trays, some of it—and I think knowing what they already know gives you your starting point. Hearing what they recount to you compared to what you were told they were told is also very useful to know—sort of cognitively and emotionally what they're able to understand at the time. And then I sort of frame my discussion from there.

There are some people who are information gatherers and they listen to everything people say, they retain everything people say, they know that they have cancer, and they just want to hear the specifics and what we're going to do about it. Other people are still a little bit disbelieving and so then you sort of have to start with the data. You know, "Here's what we saw when we looked under the microscope. This is… this is what it is," and kind of go from there.

Some doctors choose to talk to the parents and child together, while others talk to parents separately first and then talk with the child later. Some think it's important to have an ancillary relative present, such as an aunt or uncle, to serve as backup if the parents become too emotionally overwhelmed and unable to process further information. This also provides another frame of reference for discussion when the family is left alone after hearing the news.

One doctor's strategy is to tell everyone together:

> Generally I never tell the parents without the kid in the room... Some families say, "Oh, don't tell." Kids usually are way ahead of the parents. A two-year-old may not know he has cancer nor what that means but he knows he's got a lump or he's got something and he doesn't feel well. For the most part the kid's imagination is way worse than reality. Even though when you're talking to parents you may use words that a three-year-old may not understand. A seventeen-year-old will.
>
> It's still... they don't get as worried about what you might be telling mommy about what's going on if they're there. They can tune it out; it's fairly easy for any of the kids—to hand them a toy or something—to get them engaged elsewhere.
>
> I usually never do it [without someone besides the parents and child] either... Most of the time the first time you go through it with the families it doesn't all sink in. It's helpful to have another pair of ears. Then when someone doesn't remember, another person can be like, "Oh no, I was there. This is exactly what they said," kind of thing.

Other pediatric oncologists offer what is called a "warning shot" in medicine. It consists of some phrase or introductory setup that lets the family know a serious issue will be discussed next in the conversation. This way, they are able to emotionally prepare as much as possible. It can be as simple as, "we need to talk about some bad news now" or hinting by asking, "is there someone else you or your son/daughter want in the room for our discussion?" All of these phrases precede bad news. A similar sentiment is conveyed when doctors schedule this discussion to occur in a formal setting such as a conference or family meeting room.

Some physicians personalize their message to include specific points regarding the patient's diagnosis. Here's one oncologist who stresses to every family that cancer is no one's fault and this is something that can be treated:

> My essentials of my first meeting with people, there are two things that I try to get across to them... One is, "This is not your fault. Nothing you did or didn't do caused your child to have cancer." Depending on the developmental capacity of the patient, lots of kids in the school-age-group or the younger ones still have a little bit of magical thinking. So, they think the whole world revolves around them and that everything that happens is their fault. So, a lot of times I'll try to sort of take the wind out of those sails right away.

> But every single parent thinks that this is their fault. So I always just say it out loud

so they hear it. And I usually tell the mom, "Nothing you ate when you were pregnant and nothing you did." The relief on their faces is overwhelming. I always say it out loud.

The second of the key points is that, "This is something we can do something about," unless of course, it's not. But, for the most part in pediatric oncology, you can do something about it. So those are my main two points… if they don't learn anything else from that first conversation, they should learn, "It's not your fault and this is something we can do something about."

The rest is details.

Another doctor interestingly used those exact words, "we can do something", when describing his method:

My approach has always been to be very direct and honest with the family and the patient, but also, give it as gently as possible. Of course, it's one of the worst things you could hear as a parent. Although, at the onset, I always feel like that conversation is not the worst. At least at that point, you can always say that, "Your child has cancer," or "You have cancer," depending on the age of the patient, "but we can do something about it."

These conversations take time. All doctors agreed that this first conversation demands ample time:

> I think once you get into it, you really sort of let parents know and then give them time. It's to process that. I don't put any time limits on my conversations like this at all. One thing I always tell all my parents is, "You don't leave until I've answered all your questions. If I can't answer them, I will find the answers and set up a plan to get back to you with them."

Another oncologist described it as:

> When you have your first day talk like that... we will reserve a ton of time. This set-up is not like a medical office where it's like, okay, you've got fifteen minutes to see two patients. It's like no, you've got a list of patients and each one is going to get all the time that they need.

The above approach causes tension in the lives of pediatric oncologists as sometimes they prioritize their patients' needs over their outside of medicine lives. This approach offers patients and families the time and counsel they desperately need in this field. It is commonplace for providers to stay in the hospital through the dinner hour, go home to their families to put their own kids to bed, and resume writing clinical notes into the late hours of the night only to repeat the next day.

This doctor shared a similar sentiment about time:

> You have to sort of plan on spending at least an hour with the family during that first conversation. It's always setting aside, getting rid of your pager, getting rid of anything else and just making sure that you have dedicated time to spend with them. It can be difficult, especially that first conversation, because it seems like it's always the middle of the night and the family is exhausted. For them it's a very difficult time to hear, not just difficult news, but just because of the whole situation.

Here is the overall approach from one doctor's point of view. He describes the telling of a cancer diagnosis in two parts. One is the "we think this is cancer" segment and the second is "we know this is cancer" segment. He describes both:

> There are two steps; the first part is the, "We think you have cancer," or, "We think your child has cancer." That's often taking place in the emergency room or late at night in a brand new admission. I often don't do that anymore myself, but I did that a ton as a fellow. You're meeting families for the first time and saying, "We're worried that this is leukemia." Then the second part is once you've confirmed the diagnosis, you know the plan, and how you're going to

move forward from there. It's a little bit different depending on each encounter, obviously, and on the age of the patient.

For the first type of encounter, where we think the child might have cancer, I usually will have that conversation with the parents. I'll say we have a strong suspicion, this is why, and we basically need to do additional tests to really figure out what's going on. For an older teenager, I will include them in that conversation. For a younger child, I think it can be too confusing, stressful, and too involved to really bring that up in an initial pass unless we know that it's cancer.

Then the second part is once you've confirmed the diagnosis and you know the plan and how you're going to move forward from there. For the second type of conversation, it is again age dependent. For older teenagers, I'll have one meeting where I include parents, caregivers, and the older teen. For younger patients, I do it separately and have one meeting with the parents. Then at the end of that meeting, I say, "Now we have to go talk with Johnny. We have to talk with him about what's going on in language that he will understand." Some families like to have that conversation alone with their child, in which case I can give them some suggested words—how to explain it and talking points to try to hit that we want to reinforce. Or I tell them, "We are happy to do this with you, in your presence."

I think it's 50/50; half the parents say, "Please do it for me," and half the parents say, "No, we want to do this in private, thank you very much." That's the setting for how we do this.

In terms of the words that I use, for the family meeting, I use a very outlined approach of what I need to cover during that meeting. I need to let them know what the diagnosis is, what the treatment is, and what the prognosis is. Somewhere along the line what the cause is or what we believe the cause might be for the cancer. The corollary to that is that it's not something that the child did or the parents did or something along those lines.

I tend to be very direct and say, "We know what this is. We've done all the tests. This is leukemia, that is a form of cancer," and get that out of the way. We usually try to have breaks in between each of those subsections where we talk about what the diagnosis is and then ask if there are questions or things that

> they're not understanding, then talk
> about the treatment, ask if there are
> questions, and then talk about the
> prognosis and ask if there are questions.

Another's strategy is to make sure everyone starts with a simple understanding of the biology:

> It's starting with the most basic thing. If
> it's a new leukemia diagnosis I start with
> what's in blood and what are the normal
> blood cells. Because most of these kids
> show up anemic [low red blood cells]
> and thrombocytopenic [low platelets] so
> that is part of the discussion anyway.
> Most of these people don't have a sense
> as to what leukemia is. They know it's a
> cancer but that's about it. I work through
> step-wise what the diagnosis is. If they
> don't get that first sense of it, then
> everything else is going to be more
> difficult for them to understand.

Like a well-staged drama, the script is not the only important piece to have fluent and organized beforehand. Equally important as what is being said is how that information is being said. Here's another doctor's approach that highlights the strategy of sitting down to convey accessibility and commonality with the family and child:

> Obviously one of the more important
> things actually when you come into a
> room you sit down, you try to sit down
> because perhaps it makes you more

approachable and lets the family know that you are going to be there for a little bit to address their concerns. That is something I always do. I also initially get a sense of what brought them to the hospital first; let them tell me their story about how they ended up here, whether it is in the emergency room or in our clinic. I just try to listen and gauge from the parents how to approach the diagnosis because in a lot of ways, a lot of them already have a suspicion. It's basically up to you to just confirm that suspicion. A lot of them perhaps have already been told by their primary care physician about the possibilities, but some of them have no idea whatsoever. So in those patients, you kind of have to walk them through it a little bit more.

And once we get that done, maybe try to do a physical exam and pay attention to what the parents say, what brought their child to medical attention. Really sit down after that with them and tell them what we found out with the labs. For leukemia, I say, well I noticed that your child's white count is elevated and that's concerning. At that point, bring up the term leukemia or you know, sarcoma or something like that, and ask if they know what that is. Some of them do, certainly. And most everybody knows that it is some form of cancer. In general, I don't avoid the term cancer, some people perhaps do. But I think that if you're using the term leukemia, they do have to understand that it is a cancer. So, a lot of them will ask if that's a cancer and I say yes it is a cancer. So I kind of bring it out right there.

But you try to individualize it. You certainly do because pretty much at that point they will start crying, and they may not hear anything else you say. In which case you have to let them cry and get it out and usually some individual will start asking questions. Usually it is the dads, they seem to be much more empirical I think. And they will start to ask, "how can you be sure?" or like, "what makes you think this is the case?" and a lot of them will almost immediately move on to, "what's next?", "how did we diagnose this?", or "how do we make sure?", those types of questions. For the parents who aren't as cognizant of what leukemia is, I try to explain to them about the bone marrow. If it is a sarcoma or a solid tissue tumor like osteosarcoma or Ewing's sarcoma, I say to them, "there are some abnormal cells". So I try to explain that to them a little bit.

Besides explaining his rationale for sitting with the family, the above doctor also intentionally tries to use the word cancer. That one word has the ability to conjure such a multitude of feelings. Perhaps more than any other diagnosis, cancer has developed its own identity to the point of embodying lifelike though haunting characteristics. It can swiftly invoke feelings of fear, shock, death, evil, or denial in an individual during a single usage. In describing the initial diagnosis, almost all doctors seem to believe that parents need to understand they are dealing with cancer. In subsequent conversations, other words and phrases are thrown around as if to attempt to avoid the emotional response that the word cancer evokes. Substitutive words include malignancy, tumor, mass, blast, or abnormal cells. Unfortunately, while these linguistic maneuvers may be well intentioned, they create confusion, which should be avoided above all else in a discussion already inherently confusing. The shock alone creates enough formidable barriers to patient and parent understanding. Here are one doctor's thoughts on the word cancer and the ensuing emotional upheaval it inflicts after hearing it:

> I think it's pretty straightforward. I usually say the results that we have back show that you have cancer, and that it's this particular thing. I think I always use the word cancer, and I always use the actual name of the diagnosis. I often use those specific terms with the kid too but it may come with more explanation depending on what they need.

When talking with pediatric patients, some doctors admit that they tend to avoid using the word cancer initially. One physician attempts to shield his younger patients despite recognizing this approach is a bit absurd given kids will eventually understand and identify their diagnosis with the word cancer:

> I always use the word tumor unless the family has decided that they don't even want the child to know that he or she has that. Yet they're not unintelligent children; they can read and see that they're coming to the [redacted] Cancer Center, or they see [redacted] Hospital for Cancer on the front of the building. They can look stuff up on the web.

> I'll generally use the word tumor. It really will, then, I think, vary with age exactly how much I tell the kids. There is honestly no methodology for it. It's not like I say, okay, well if they're this age, I do that. This next group, I do that... you know, you really just have to adjust. Because I've worked with seven-year-olds who are going on thirty, and I've worked with fifteen-year-olds who are going on six.

In the beginning, the initial innate parental response is to become hyper-protective. Parents sometimes jump to a conclusion that the best tactic to protect their children from distress is to not tell them they have cancer. Not only is this strategy difficult to maintain, almost all pediatric oncologists were wholly against this practice. It doesn't encourage the child to share feelings about their illness when the surrounding adults are abstaining from discussing it. Below are some thoughts from doctors on how they tailor their discussion based upon age and how they approach parents to convince them to tell the child about his or her cancer:

> Usually for kids... most kids that are thirteen or fourteen or so, by this time I would have already felt out the family to get of sense of how much they're comfortable with the kid knowing up front. Often I will be told, "We don't want them to know anything." I won't necessarily accept that at face value. I think the kid eventually needs to know. I will respect it up front in the sense that I will have the conversation first with the family. Obviously, a one year old does not really... You can have it in the same room because they do not really understand everything anyway.
>
> Other kids, age four to ten or so, I will have the family separately. I'll tell them that at some point we should describe the diagnosis to the child. I'll tell them in a separate meeting, which is usually very long and involved. I like to very clearly lay out what the diagnosis is, what the general prognosis is, what the treatment plan is. At some point I'll say that I feel strongly that we need to communicate some of this to your child. Except for very rare circumstances, they will be in agreement with that.

Not only is it important intellectually for a child to come to terms with his or her diagnosis, but the initial response and eventual emotional transition depends largely on having the correct and complete information. For one oncologist, all kids should know what's going on at some level so they can begin to emotionally cope with it.

> I think it depends on the level of understanding of the child. If the kid developmentally is above the age of, I don't know, seven, eight, or nine, they will have heard the word cancer before but they may not understand it on a biologic basis. But it's important that they know and they have a name for what they have so that they can sort of think it through. But also when their friends ask them, "What do you have?" they can tell them.

> But for little kids, you know, three, four, or five, it can be, "There's something in your body that shouldn't be there and we're going to make it better." But whether you call it cancer or not, I don't know that they can understand that at that age.

For adolescents, oncologists had a slightly different approach. Doctors seek to be clear about the diagnosis with them, but some convey this information with intentional ambiguity concerning prognosis, especially if it is a cancer with poor outcomes. This doctor relays that he doesn't like most children or adolescents to initially know if they have a cancer that is likely to result in death:

> In an older child, and that can be an eight, ten, or twelve year old, then usually we try to go into a little bit more detail of why they are here and a little bit more detail of what we expect in terms of their hospital stay and procedures. We reassure them that the procedures are done under anesthesia, they won't feel anything, and to expect that ...

> In older children, a fifteen, sixteen, or seventeen year old, obviously you tell them what the diagnosis is, because if you don't tell them, they will find out very soon from the internet. You tell them, and you give an explanation, a general plan of what the therapy will be like, what the change in their routines will be. Usually in the beginning, myself, I always give an optimistic sense to them.

> I mean I usually don't feel like I need to tell them exactly what is happening with their health then. Unless we are talking, unless it is with somebody older, a twenty-four year old, or things like that, then maybe. More close to what the odds actually are, or definitely closer.

This doctor, like most, tells parents that he would never lie to a child. When all is said and done, the supremacy of the doctor-patient relationship, the most important bond of trust in medicine, prevails even in pediatrics. In pediatrics, that the patient happens to be a child is not irrelevant, but does not change the fundamental tenet that a doctor's first loyalty is to his or her patient. Thus, the child's questions and fears deserve addressing, even in situations where answering would fly in the face of the parents' wishes. One doctor asserts that he always tells children the truth when they ask a question:

> The one tangent on that would be that occasionally parents feel very strongly that they want to protect their child from the diagnosis and they don't want us to use the word cancer or tumor or something. It may vary about how they feel about that, and what I always try to tell them is it's probably impossible, really, to keep the child from that, if they're old enough that they're literate kids, they're coming to the [redacted] Cancer Center.

> The other kids they're talking to in the play room are all talking about their cancers, so it's probably impossible to keep that from them. I think it's not a good idea in any case, because it creates an awkward dynamic between the child and the parents, where there's something that's not supposed to be said, that maybe the child wants to talk about.

> So, that can be an awkward thing at
> certain points. Of course usually we try
> to compromise and reach some happy
> medium with the parents. One thing I
> always tell the parents is that I would
> never lie to the child, so if the child asks
> me a question, I'm always going to
> answer it honestly, taking into account,
> of course their developmental status. I
> may not tell them the entire truth but
> certainly, I'm not going to tell them an
> untruth if they ask me a question.

Yet, the child is not the only person with whom uncomfortable truths should not be hidden. Cancer is a deadly disease. Children die from cancer and unfortunately, they can die from both the "good" cancers (cancers with cure rates around 90%) as well as from the "bad" cancers (cancers where cure rates are less than 50%). Therefore, during that initial, day one discussion, some oncologists think it is important to explicitly state that cancer is life threatening. Telling parents their child may die from this disease, especially when the doctor has only met them that day, is quite the undertaking for both parties – the doctor and the parents. Yet some physicians feel quite strongly that the possibility needs to be communicated. This is one of those doctors talking about prognosis and the need to be upfront about the possibility of death:

> I think I usually do a combination of
> numbers and then something that's more
> conceptual. I always start every
> conversation saying this is a life
> threatening illness, that at least… at

some point in the discussion, we have to acknowledge that dying from the disease is a possibility. We don't have to dwell on it. We don't have to make it the focus of our attention but it's on the table as a possibility. Because I think that… parents, I think different parents hear that in different ways or choose to.

I can't really think of any cancer in which at some point in time, it's not a possibility. I feel like it's sort of a disservice if we don't acknowledge the severity of what we're dealing with. Sometimes I think also it's important because you're setting the stage for saying the treatment that is coming forward is going to be really hard and tough, but the consequences of not doing it are really life-threatening.

This is an important idea to convey; parents need to understand this is a serious diagnosis and, although human nature makes us reticent to vocalize it, part of the doctor's responsibility is to make sure parents understand the full gravity of the situation and the necessity of adhering to treatment.

My goal for the person is for them to understand the diagnosis and understand, not necessarily percentage-wise but the severity of it. Have some sense of prognosis and what the therapy entails. With most of the diagnoses here

> part of the prognosis includes the fact
> that this is something that could be fatal.
> Your child may die of this.

Conversely, a provider's intent is not to crush all hope. It is a delicate balancing act between gloom and optimism, wherein each idea put forth conveys a certain tone and pushes the mood of the conversation one direction or the other. With manipulation and clinical expertise, doctors can be honest, upfront, and inspire hope. One encounter I witnessed was a twenty-two-year-old man coming into the clinic with his mother after having a warm, painful, and swollen knee for weeks. Two different hospitals had told him to take ibuprofen for a presumed case of severe arthritis. Yet, an eventual magnetic resonance imaging (MRI) scan revealed a tumor, following which a needle biopsy showed a type of solid cancer called osteosarcoma. The mother and son were made aware of the cancer diagnosis before arriving at the oncology clinic for an appointment. At this point, the pediatric oncologist has gathered the history and performed a physical in which he stated to me, as the medical student, that the knee was "very impressive" which is code for striking or interesting. In this case, the knee was noticeably warm because of the tumor. He also walked the patient and his mother through the MRI scan, calling the cancerous tumor a "bright spot" when pointing to it on the screen. Both were interesting word choices. What follows is how the physician conveyed the seriousness of this "good cancer".

> Doctor: This cancer is treatable and the
> chances are promising; there is a 90%
> chance everything will be fine. I'm a
> straight shooter; I'll tell it like it is.

Mom: I appreciate that.

Doctor: You have a serious problem. What it is and where it is are both concerning. In cases like these, there is a 65-70% chance of long term disease management or cure as it's non-metastatic *[Then he explained chemotherapy for nine to ten months, the process of putting in a portovac (medication access route under the skin), treatment with surgery, as well as enrolling in a clinical trial to add more agents to see "if there's a way to do better."]*

Doctor: This is a hard, but doable road. Any questions?

Patient: Does chemo hurt? Will I be able to live a normal life after all is done?

Doctor: *[After answering questions]* Lots of times people hear cancer and they think they're dead. I want to make sure that you know that this isn't a death sentence.

Mom: *[to me afterward]* I knew it would be a rough conversation, but I didn't know how rough it would be.

Words are important, especially in this initial encounter where the goal is to lay the foundation for trust and understanding upon which to build a successful treatment plan. In the above conversation, many technical and medical terms littered the doctor's speech. These can impede parent and patient understanding. Even concrete numbers, statistics, and probabilities can be confusing if the full context of that data is not entirely understood. What does "a 90% chance everything will be fine" or "a 65-70% chance of long term disease management or cure" mean? There were a lot of technical and medical words in the above conversation. It did not seem to me the mother or the patient understood all of it. In looking back, I'm still confused as to what the doctor meant by the percentages that he gave.

Increasing the potential for misunderstanding is the limit on time. Most physicians do not have ample opportunity to expound for lengthy periods to explain complex concepts; as shown by the brevity in his above responses and explanations. The most impressive doctors are able to accomplish many goals and transfer comprehensible information in a brief amount of time, while never appearing rushed. This is a skill that can be learned and taught to a degree, but also one that comes more naturally to some - in style, composition, and in fostering understanding.

Each doctor, whether they are conscious of it or not, has a style in how they disclose a cancer diagnosis as unique as the physician himself.

> I think when it comes time to actually sit
> and tell the parents, I don't... maybe I
> have a style, maybe somebody would
> have to watch me and tell me what my
> style is. You know you're not giving
> them good news. It could be what to me
> is relatively good, meaning I'm telling
> you that you have a tumor that we have a
> lot of success in treating versus I'm

telling you that we have a tumor that is more of a challenge for us to treat versus I'm telling you that overall there's one tumor type that we take care of where the 1-year survival ranks in the single digits.

I do have to tailor it a little bit. You're not giving good news, so I think you have to be clear. You really have to think about what you're saying and the language in which you're saying it.

Honestly, I'm very lucky that the bulk of my friends are very intelligent, and when we talk, we have intelligent conversations and words are polysyllabic. But, sometimes you have to think about what these families... Okay, this is not a family that has had those educational opportunities, so you have to change the wording of what you're saying. You have to be mindful so that they understand what you are saying. You have to check that they understand.

Repeatedly gauging understanding is a conversational clinical tactic to make sure the physician is not talking over the heads of his or her patients. This strategy could have produced more comprehension in the prior-mentioned conversation between the oncologist and the twenty-two-year-old with osteosarcoma. Although time consuming, it is very effective. While that doctor may not have had the time to do this in his busy oncology practice, it is a strategy that should be employed whenever possible balancing other constraints. Verifying comprehension ensures that the patient remains the focus of clinical medicine.

These conversations are difficult to have. They are rich in emotional depth and breadth, and yet they become routine for a pediatric oncologist. It is hard to believe that you would get used to such a transformative, emotional conversation in which you tell someone else they have cancer, but it does happen. Here one oncologist reflects on remembering to remain sensitive:

> We've seen hundreds of new patients. We, as this patient's oncologist, have been through this hundreds of times, but this is their first, hopefully, only time they ever have to go through this.
>
> It's very easy to get crass as you're going through this process. You see so many new patients... you can kind of get thinking like "the new leukemia in the such and such room" instead of thinking like "John who is a four year old child in the midst of a difficult situation, the parents recently divorced, and all these kinds of things". You really need to understand the background of the family and their level of understanding of the disease process; and then I tailor it to that.

Routine might seem ill advised in this setting, but paradoxically it can be beneficial for perfecting a framework in which to disclose a cancer diagnosis as long as it's tailored to the patient's specific circumstances each time. With each successive conversation, doctors learn better and more effective techniques to add to their repertoire. Over years seeing hundreds of patient and families, they can anticipate questions and have experienced the majority of possible reactions. They've dealt with angry parents, the crying child, grief-stricken siblings, silence, shock, and all other possible combinations. Having been part of the process more than once, they are better able to anticipate and address the responses in subsequent occasions.

One of the fundamental responsibilities of any pediatric oncologist is to break bad news to patients and families. By the time they have come through fellowship and "into their own" as an attending, they have done it countless times. In many ways, they have become accustomed to their roles and each has written a different script that fits their particular style and which they can recite automatically. While their communication techniques are rooted in compassion, this is a conversation that needs to relay medical and practical information. The goal is always understanding—of the diagnosis, treatment, and prognosis—for all involved. It's an arduous task to tell a family and patient of a new cancer diagnosis. At the same time, the difficulty of the task does not preclude the experienced physician from being able to exude confidence and competence while inspiring hope, comprehension, and trust.

That moment when the doctor discloses the diagnosis to the patient and family unifies all those involved. It is a common thread that runs through all patient stories about cancer. In some ways, it separates them from those in the general population who have never had to personally come to terms with this information about themselves or their children. Learning of a cancer diagnosis provokes unique feelings and begins a mental transformation that few can comprehend. That conversation is the beginning of a journey.

CHAPTER 8

Trust

"The treatment of a disease may be entirely impersonal; the care of the patient must be completely personal. The significance of the intimate personal relationship between physician and patient cannot be too strongly emphasized, for in an extraordinarily large number of cases both diagnosis and treatment are directly dependent on it."

—Francis Weld Peabody, *The Care of the Patient*

Trust is a unifying force. Typically, its strength is forged through deliberate effort over time. In medicine, however, this emotion can bypass this formidable course to take a faster route. It develops in the doctor-patient relationship with little buildup or effort, simply expected by both sides. This trust must be sustained both in situations of intense stress and in spite of large gaps in power and knowledge.

The trust that exists within the doctor-patient relationship may be more fragile and fleeting than if it had developed over time. One misstep by either party may destroy trust just as quickly as it was created. Sadly, it is one of the most irrecoverable of qualities; once it is lost, it almost never returns. Doctors are acutely aware of this finicky nature as they navigate their patient and family relationships. They know the value in trust to attain accurate information and to guide treatment decisions.

A trusting relationship is a fruitful one for both the provider and patient. In its absence, all suffer. Teams function through trust, and medicine is a team endeavor. In pediatric oncology, the players are doctors, nurses, social workers, child life specialists, techs, family members, and of course, the patient. For the healthcare process to function smoothly, all members must work together where every person knows and executes his or her role. This is best accomplished in an environment of respect and trust. As a medical student, I felt inspired when I realized the level of trust that is given to us as healthcare professionals. It took only a few patients to realize the enormity of this responsibility and the gravity of it as a gift. In wearing that white coat as a medical student, I was automatically trusted by my patients and their families. They answered my invasive questions about intimate details of their lives and gave me access to examine their bodies. All was well intentioned and in pursuit of providing the best care, but this is still such a unique and remarkable practice. Conferring that level of trust to complete strangers based solely upon their profession is a peculiar practice. With this in mind, doctors must learn how to best use the trust that is given, as it's one of the most powerful tools in their arsenal. They depend on it to gather accurate diagnostic information, affect decision making, and influence health behavior both inside and outside the hospital.

To artfully tell and explain a new cancer diagnosis to a child and family requires tact and skill. It is a conversation that not only transfers information, but it also builds a relationship. In many instances, the initial encounter is this conversation. Thus, the family and patient meet their supervising oncologist when they are hearing about a new cancer diagnosis for the first time. The physician who makes the diagnosis will often be assigned to that patient throughout the treatment course. This relationship will develop over many subsequent inpatient and outpatient encounters, but its foundation is laid during that first conversation. Oncologists take much ownership of their patients, and this initial meeting sets the stage for that connection. It is therefore important that the doctor gets it right. One doctor believes that the first conversation is the most important opportunity to develop that trusting relationship:

> The thing you're really trying to establish in the first meeting is what I call therapeutic alliance, where you're trying to basically form a trust relationship. All of medicine is relationship based... A huge part of that first meeting is establishing trust. When we have that first conversation with the family, there's no other time like it as far as having this point of trust building.

> To establish that therapeutic alliance, there are three main things I really focus on. The first point is understanding what they're going through. So, trying my very best to empathize with them. It's trying to empty myself of preconceived notions of how other people have been before them and how they received the

information. It is to say, "Okay, where are you at? What do you know? What's the best way to communicate with you?" It's trying to really understand who they are.

In understanding that, I try to look at what their values are, what their hopes and fears are. I look at things like, "What are you most worried about? What is it now that you know what's going on? What is it that you're most hopeful for?" That's the first step. It's an understanding piece from their perspective.

The second point is sharing relevant information. Meaning, "What information do they need right now? What is it that is a barrier to them before they move forward?" Some people... the information they need is in depth information about their disease process. Some people, what they need is just simply saying, "Most kids with this can be cured." As soon as you say that, they're like, "Okay." You're not lying to them. You're just going to tell them something that is a piece of information that's clearly prohibiting them from moving forward. It's either in the relationship or their understanding of what's going on. That is a step that I call sharing relevant information.

The kids with brain tumors, it's going over their MRI [imaging scan] results with them. When you walk in the room and you have the MRI results, no one would sit there and ask them, "What is it that you're most concerned about today?" That is a big mistake. You want to tell them the MRI results or share this relevant information.

The third step to relationship building and having this conversation go in the right way is understanding their needs from their perspective. Not me coming in and saying, "This is what you need." But me listening and figuring out from their perspective what they need. Every family is unique. Every family-physician interaction is unique. Every relationship between family and the physician is unique. You can't come in and just perform the FICA spirituality assessment [a standardized assessment tool about faith]. Yeah, you want to come in there maybe do a spiritual assessment like that, but you want to also really understand what it means... their responses and contexts within that particular family.

Each physician seemed to have a particular strategy to develop a trusting relationship quickly and deeply. Many of them draw on their extensive experience with similar situations. After guiding hundreds of patients and families through a cancer diagnosis and treatment experience, a pediatric oncologist is able to develop lots of strategies in relationship building. One seasoned physician draws on this experience to develop trust and portray confidence:

> When people tell me what they're experiencing, I now have pretty much heard it before and can give them that reassurance. Not so much that I trivialize what they are saying, but by saying that I've heard this a thousand times and I have more sense of how to go through it. From my time in medical school — which is when I learned how to talk to people about this — it has become easier to feel comfortable. I hope to be able to exude that sense of confidence that they will make the best decision for themselves and for their child and for them to truly feel that.

Trust is one of those sentiments that you cannot fully appreciate until it's gone. Once it leaves the doctor-patient relationship, it is difficult to compassionately and effectively deliver healthcare. Medicine depends on trust. Diagnosis and symptom management depend on information supplied by the patient and family. But most importantly, successful decision making and care function only if the patient and family trust the opinion and knowledge of the physician enough to follow his or her lead. In pediatrics, it is rare to have an unproductive relationship, but it does happen. I have seen it falter from both sides — the patient and the provider — and this destroys the trust environment. Some of the most tenuous relationships have revolved around managing pain as a symptom. Pain is deeply complex in its biological, psychological, and social roots. As doctors cannot objectively measure a patient's pain level, there can be differences of opinion in management and appropriate drug treatment. Opiates, a class of medicine whose active ingredient is similar to the active ingredient in heroin, are highly effective; yet, they pose the risk for maladaptive use, abuse, and even addiction. They are rarely a long-term solution, but do provide benefits in many acute pain crises.

As the acute pain subsides, physicians seek to wean patients off of these medicines and transition them to better-targeted regimens. Yet, some patients do not want to be weaned. Pain is a subjective experience, and we do not have perfect medications for every situation. The most difficult situations occur with adolescent patients, with those who struggle with chronic pain, and with those who develop an addiction to pain medications. For example, I have witnessed screaming matches where patients are arguing for continuation of pain medicines to anyone who will listen. Some strongly desire pain medication via intravenous (IV) route, which while faster, delivers some version of a "rush". When providers are reluctant to give these kinds of pain medicines, it erodes patient trust and simultaneously reduces physicians' confidence in their patients. Doctors may feel these patients have ulterior motives and are not seeking treatment based purely on pain-driven reasons. This is a totally destructive process leading to diminished trust in the healthcare system.

To illustrate this point, consider the story of one twenty-five-year-old woman who survived cancer, but was left with chronic pain that eroded her trust in the medical system. When she was eleven years old, she was diagnosed with osteosarcoma, a type of soft tissue tumor, of her right femur. During that year, she had a surgical resection of the tumor, underwent chemotherapy, and was fitted for a leg prosthesis. At thirteen, she suffered a relapse meaning her cancer came back, and it spread to her lungs and involved her hip. At fifteen, she received a hip replacement. Now, almost a decade later at age twenty-five, she lives with cancer as a chronic disease. For her, cure is unlikely and the prosthesis, hip replacement, and multiple drug side effects have left her with chronic pain of her joints and bones. She follows up at the pain clinic, a specialized center for patients who deal with complex and significant pain. Yet, she has not seen a provider or scheduled an appointment in many months even though she suffers from considerable pain on a daily basis. Here is the exchange I witnessed between her and the doctor:

> Doctor: Why didn't you come earlier?

> Patient: Pain is all I've known. The past two years have been tough. Other people look at me and can't be bothered.

> Doctor: Don't know if it's that, it could be that they don't want to do any damage.

As I looked at this woman who was in so much physical pain, I was struck by the fact that her emotional pain seemed even greater. She looked reluctant to be there and appeared afraid that everyone was judging her. Echoed through her words, she conveyed her loss of trust and faith in her doctors. She thought they couldn't be "bothered" with her. This deterioration of trust is a tragedy and a failing of the medical system. It has clearly caused her much pain, both in the literal physical and emotional sense. The "damage" has already been done.

Another situation which destroys trust is when some decision makers do not want the doctor to share information with certain parties. This is commonly seen when parents do not want their child to know an aspect of the disease or its course, such as that they have cancer or that they are going to die as curative treatment has failed. Doctors often feel strongly that the child has the right to know. But when parents disagree, it presents a choice point. Trust is easily lost between providers and parents in these situations if not handled carefully. Do the parents' wishes supersede the child's right to know about his or her body and impending death? Is this dependent on age? Which trust relationship is valued most in this situation, the doctor-parent or the doctor-patient relationship? Here are one doctor's thoughts:

> We'll come up with some sort of strategy as to how you want to tell them and what words to use. For four to twelve, we'll sit down and say something like, "You're very sick," or using the word cancer or leukemia or whatever it is. I personally strive to get as truthful as the family will let me with the child without burning bridges. It's always easy to say, "Well, the child has to know." But, you have to take into account what bridges you might burn if you go against the family's wishes in something like that. In general, I don't do that.
>
> Kids above that I'll insist that they hear

at some point what we're doing and why
we're doing it. I will push for all of those
kids to know… at some point.

Another doctor describes a situation in which he was unable
to have a full conversation with a seventeen year old patient
about death because her father didn't want his daughter, the
patient, to know she was dying of her osteosarcoma:

> I will have already talked with the family
> out of the room, and say this is what I
> want to tell them. I will strive to be very
> honest with them. I generally don't find
> at the end of the day it's worth it to burn
> bridges if families say, "We don't want
> you to tell her that." I had a seventeen
> year old patient that died of metastatic
> osteosarcoma where I knew she knew
> what was going on, but the dad would
> never actually let me tell her that. I
> would gently push each time I saw them
> to let me talk honestly with her. If I'm
> allowed to then, yes, I will tell them.

This physician believed he was still able to have a fulfilling
relationship even though he was unable to openly discuss her
prognosis with her. In reflecting upon this, he even relayed
that she was one of his favorite patients:

> The most involved I was with a family
> was a patient who unfortunately died of
> osteosarcoma. She had a lot of ups and
> downs from being a fairly positive
> prognosis, non metastatic osteosarcoma,

to having an extensive lymph salvage procedure, and then later having a late relapse and going through a number of medicines. The dad was very intense and wanted to continue therapy...

I wasn't able to really successfully get him to allow me to tell her her prognosis. I got to know the family and girl very well, and I liked her very much. I just cared for her very much. I invested a huge amount of time and energy, and I do think that at the end I was able to help them meet goals with regard to her dying at home and dying relatively comfortably at home, which is really not easy to arrange. So, I do feel gratified at being involved in her care. I think the family reciprocated that, so I guess she stands out as a favorite. She was seventeen when she died, maybe thirteen when she was diagnosed. It was a long course.

Another physician commented:

Honestly this is a much more of an issue than it is something that comes up frequently because people make it a bigger issue than it really needs to be. But you need to be on the side of the parents. You need to align with them. After aligning with them, then you can encourage them to do the right thing.

> The place people get in trouble all the
> time is they draw lines in the sand and
> say, "I don't care what you say as a
> parent. This kid needs to know." That's
> never going to be received well. You
> really have to align with the parents.
> Then as you build that relationship you
> can be more pressing in saying, "We
> really have to have this conversation with
> your child." But if you come in and just
> do it, the relationship is over. They will
> probably fire you actually and stuff.

If the doctor patient relationship is not working out
for many reasons or trust is not developing, patients or
families may "fire" a doctor. This means they refuse to see a
certain physician or allow him or her to participate in the
child's care; they will be reassigned to a different primary
physician. "Being fired" means that the family or patient
demands that you not be their doctor anymore. Medicine at
its core is still a service industry and in that, the patient
functions as a pseudo consumer. One can imagine that for a
professional with good intentions and much experienced
training, this can be very personally insulting and painful.
Occasionally, trust does not develop between patients and
providers. Sometimes the reason is not clear and it remains
unknown what went wrong. A physician recounted an
encounter with a patient when she was an intern, she had
finished medical school and was the most junior doctor on
the team:

> Internship is tough and when you don't
> make exactly the right choice, people can
> really get down on you... I remember

one patient who had liver disease. Nobody knew why he had liver disease. He wasn't getting better, and I remember as an intern I said to the attending you know, we haven't gotten I think it was an ultrasound, I remember this was like forty years ago we didn't have CAT scans, we didn't have MRIs and I said there's something going on with the liver and we had done some plain films before and didn't see anything.

And so finally they got I think it was an ultrasound and this kid had a big massive cyst. And once they identified that and went in and drained it, he began to get better. In the midst of all this, something happened with not the kid, but his father. His father said that he didn't want me taking care of his son. And I had no idea where that came from. I remember being so hurt because I was thinking to myself, "You don't understand, if I hadn't pushed for the ultrasound he wouldn't be getting better."

But that was so irrelevant to whatever the emotionality was. Whatever he had picked up from me, the father, like I said not the kid but the father was saying, "You will not come in here again." It just seemed so unfair. Wait a minute, I found the problem.

So internship's a tough time and being able to maintain your sense of self and to truly believe throughout that entire experience that you really are doing the best that you can and that you're always working in the best interest of the patient. That gets challenged over and over again. So I would say that was the depths of despair that year. It got better being a resident and kept going up from there.

Most physician patient bonds are strong. Partnerships form where goals, personalities, and emotions align. Pediatrics is a field known for strong personal connections. It is an immense privilege to be able to form these relationships. From my anecdotal experience and from asking doctors to name their favorite patients, it seems that the more intense the emotional situation the stronger the bond that forms. This doctor seemed to agree:

> I think some of the most important relationships that I've had with people have been patients and families at the end of life. And I feel like it has been a tremendous privilege for me. And so even though it's hard and sad, it's really enriching. You're so lucky to be there in these really intimate parts of people's lives. That sounds a little voyeuristic, but I don't intend it to be that way at all.

> I think it's a privilege that you get to be part of it.

With that privilege comes an immense requirement for trust. Imagine the level needed in this relationship as described by this doctor. It takes much trust to hold hands with your doctor as you die:

> It seems like a lot of times people die in the middle of the night or the wee hours of the morning. And I can think of far too many kids, sitting and holding their hands while they died… there's something really striking about a patient that you've known for a long time… they are sort of take-your-breath-away moments of life and you're there.

In asking physicians their thoughts on trust, many mentioned that developing a relationship requires "getting close" and there are professional and emotional challenges along the process. One doctor discusses his navigation of those boundaries and the notion of a doctor "getting too close":

> I've been asked to speak about this issue many times. I think the issue is less of boundaries than it is really truly forming this therapeutic alliance. I think that all care needs to be relationship based. To me, you need to go see that particular patient and family and give them a 100% of yourself; fully all aspects, emotionally, a 100% of who you are. Love them, form that relationship, give that to them with no expectation of anything in return, and then leave the room,

somehow shake that off and head to the next room and do the exact same thing.

Somehow I've been able to manualize things that way where I can walk into a room, give a 100% of who I am to that person in every respect... I can cry with them, I can laugh with them, I can feel completely, totally, emotionally devastated in that room giving them whatever they need. They are the focus. This is not about me. This is about them. I don't need a response from them. I don't need them to say, "We're going to get through this. It will be okay." I'm doing all this for them.

It's true emotions, but it's also not emotions with an expectation of something in return. It's also professional. Professionalism is a really critical part of this. Then somehow leaving the room, you would go wash your face, you have big tears or red eyes or whatever it is, and be able to go the next room, you do the exact same thing for that next patient.

It's different for everyone to be able to do that. I can do that a lot easier than most people because of things I went through and stuff I learned from an early age. But some people in order to do that have to actually go too far, have to cross the boundaries to see what it's like to be on the other side where they have pushed too far and gotten too close from a relationship standpoint and work turns from professional to personal.

Some of the other doctors thought that there was no such thing as becoming "too close" to a family as long as certain social boundaries were respected. Others preferred to create more of a strict line in professional boundaries. None of them seemed to think their personal strategy provided inferior emotional or medical care to their patients. They all thought they created enough space to maintain objectivity and to develop the needed trust, but they did it in many different ways.

Nurturing trust is one of the most empowering experiences in medicine. It is able to unify and support the goals of the physician, patient, and family and is vital for successful relationships. To understand its importance in healthcare requires recognizing the power and knowledge differentials in medicine. Amongst providers and patients, there is a huge gap which must be bridged through trust to best deliver healthcare. It is an idea that must be respected and cultivated by physicians. In pediatric oncology, in particular, it is of the utmost importance. Patients and families allow oncologists to enter some of the most intimate and personal spaces of their emotional lives. In children whose cancer becomes incurable, this environment is one of tremendous vulnerability, emotional depth, and at times, sadness. It's important to remember that trust is the most fragile of emotions. If its importance is forgotten or its development is ignored, trust will fade and the relationship will disintegrate. This will compromise healthcare outcomes

and provoke a shattered response in patients, families, and
doctors alike.

CHAPTER 9

Sadness
Coping with It

"Beauty and sadness always go together. Nature thought beauty too rich to go forth upon the earth without a meet alloy."

—George MacDonald

Sadness is a beast that must be contained. Those that feel or observe this emotion need to know how to control it within themselves and others. If given the power to grow unchecked, it will eventually dismantle one's sense of self. Yet, if one retains perspective and hope when immersed in sadness, one can embrace other more positive emotions even while concurrently experiencing sadness. This is important for patients, families, and doctors in pediatric oncology who exist in their respective emotional spheres. Sadness morphs into many forms throughout this field. Each time it appears, it must be fully felt and addressed in order to move beyond it. Sadness is not an emotion that can be ignored. To define this emotion and to understand its intricacies is the first step to defend against its onslaught. Yet, the key to controlling sadness is to develop a personal strategy to look it in its eye and to still charge forward with resolve and grace. That is the way doctors, patients, and families keep sadness from consuming their lives. It is a hard, but important struggle.

One of my favorite analogies describing this beautiful life philosophy is from John Green's novel, *Fault in Our Stars*. The passage is from when Hazel, the protagonist, is eulogizing her boyfriend, Augustus; both had cancer.

> There are infinite numbers between 0 and 1. There's .1 and .12 and .112 and an infinite collection of others. Of course, there is a bigger infinite set of numbers between 0 and 2, or between 0 and a million. Some infinities are bigger than other infinities. There are days, many of them, when I resent the size of my unbounded set. I want more numbers than I'm likely to get, and God, I want more numbers for Augustus Waters than he got. But, Gus, my love, I cannot tell you how thankful I am for our little infinity. I wouldn't trade it for the world. You gave me a forever within the numbered days, and I'm grateful.

I think that life is about finding our own infinities. An emotion felt can be thought of as an infinity. Whether a moment is a brief happiness during a child's last days or a prolonged joy at full recovery after tumor removal surgery, each experience is its own infinity. You could live forever in just one moment or emotion taking it for all its worth. The human experience can be that rich if you decide to frame it that way.

The beauty of pediatric oncology is found in the intricacies between the science, the illnesses, treatments, and humans experiencing it all. The power of medicine lies in the simple but profound bond between a patient and provider. This relationship is influential in offering healing to children with cancer and their families across the illness course. This is not a field where patients are diagnosed one day, undergo a short treatment course, and then are cured never to look back. It is one where treatment can last years with chemotherapy, radiation, or surgery along the way. In between, there are numerous follow-up clinic visits and hospital stays for complications. When everything is going well, a doctor can lead with comfort and ease. But when curative treatments fail, setbacks occur, or children die, a doctor needs to lead with compassion and care.

I asked pediatric oncologists about the ways they have chosen to cope with such harrowing and humbling cases. How do you cope when someone's loved one, especially a child, dies in front of your eyes? What kind of personal characteristics does it take? In their variety of answers, I found privilege served as a central theme for providers who experience a sense of fulfillment and perspective in their clinical work:

> I really think I have a God-given gift and He put my talents to use for society. I'm in the right place at the right time, and doing exactly what I'm supposed to be doing. That is incredibly reassuring because I truly feel like every day that I come here, I'm doing the right thing. I'm doing what I was put here on Earth to do. That's one response.

The other thing is what an amazing privilege it is to work in a place that gives you continual perspective. For us, you know, we frequently complain about things like, "I had a hard day at work. It's pretty difficult because I'm not getting along very well with my colleagues." Or, "I didn't get a good night rest because the kids were sick or this or that." We come to a place like this and people are dealing with life and death issues for their own children, it just gives you perspective on what really matters in life, how blessed you are. What an amazing institution this is to be able to focus on the suffering of these patients and families.

It is a real privilege to get to do what we do. The example I usually use is my brother, who is a CPA... he was an accountant and he wasn't only an accountant, he was an auditor. So, what he did is he counted what other people had already counted to make sure that they counted it right. And when I think about that, I think, "Thank God! Thank God it sometimes hurts when I'm here speaking to a patient and their family. Thank God for the emotional response that I get through my job!" It is emotionally difficult. But why would you not want your job to be an emotional struggle? Why would you want it to be bland? Here you have these highs and lows and victories and defeats. The beauty of this job is it helps you get outside of yourself. Work is usually very self-centered. Here, it feels as if your work is in outreach. Your work is trying to help other people be better, trying to help other people feel better. Very few people can say that about their jobs. Even very few people in medicine can say that about their jobs because they very frequently turn it into a business model. Pediatric oncology is a field where everyone is salaried and everyone makes the same amount of money. There is no financial incentive to go into it. So it's really a pure field.

Themes of gratitude, truth, and privilege pervade his response. He even mentions an ideological purity with a hint of distinction as compared to other fields. His statement is telling in its brutal honesty and pride. The motivations for becoming a pediatric oncologist are largely noble, but part of it is that you are doing a job that many say they could never do. You are able to cope with the sadness when others say they could not. Because of this, society bestows admiration, gratitude, and respect. Stories of children with cancer seem to invoke a unique response within society that other illnesses or fields of medicine do not. Images of bald children undergoing cancer treatment pervade in fundraising drives, media, television, and movies. Foundations like The-Make-A-Wish Foundation inspire us with tear-jerking messages of hope as they grant the wishes and dreams of children with cancer. When talking about childhood deaths, cancer springs to the forefront of our minds. This is in spite of unintentional injury and suicide being the top killers of children.

Regardless of the motivations and composition of the field, pediatric oncologists must be able to emotionally handle the weighty sadness that comes along with treating children with cancer. They have a responsibility to maintain focus in times of pressure, stress, and emotional turmoil. Acting always in patients' best interests and maintaining the composure to help guide difficult decision making is quite an undertaking. It is probably true that many doctors would not thrive in this field. The sadness and emotional range can be overwhelming for not just patients and families, but providers as well. The decision to pursue this career comes with contemplation of one's own emotional needs and deciding if the tragedy of childhood death is enough to extinguish the spark of your professional and personal identity and existence. One doctor reflects:

> For me, in my own struggle with could I
> be a pediatric oncologist, that was one of
> the things. Can I deal with patients that
> are really close to dying? I think for me,
> that answer really was yes I can. Yes it'll
> hurt, but for most of the time when
> we're seeing these patients, they're
> bubbly, active, normal acting kids who
> happen to have life threatening illnesses.

> For me, that's the thing that allows me to
> practice, the fact that the kids are still
> kids and that someone has to take care
> of these kids. Providing them with good

> palliative care and a "good death", a
> death with dignity and respect… for the
> patient and for their family, that is
> actually quite an honor to participate in
> their care in that way. You take the good
> with the bad.

Many point to participating in that emotional journey as very fulfilling no matter its outcome. In patients and families who are suffering in sadness, pediatric oncologists are greatly needed to help navigate the process. Along with the nurses, social workers, and other providers, doctors have experience in how to cope with these situations. They have participated in the care of many dying children and they are uniquely familiar with making the journey free of physical pain and full of grace.

Many oncologists felt that this field evoked an emotional response that drew them towards this specialty. The range of feelings is a regular reminder of one of the most important reasons to become a doctor: to care for patients. Such deep experiences emphasize the humanity for all involved and are able to constantly revitalize human energy within medicine. One physician talked about his motivation to remain in the field as connected to his emotional commiseration:

> I think the time when you don't feel sad
> and don't at some level feel, at least for a
> period of time, devastated on behalf of
> your patients and families, that's when
> I'm out—when I'm not sort of upset by
> it. Then it's time to get a new job.

In thinking about providers dealing with tragic situations and feelings of sadness, it's been fascinating to talk in depth with them about their experiences. I've shadowed over fifty different pediatric oncologists across the country and worked as a medical student on rotations in oncology for over two months. While my experience may be limited, my exposure during that time was broad and deep. In interacting with so many pediatric oncologists, it is my opinion that these are some of the happiest people and doctors I've ever met. How do they do it? I'm still not sure if it's just a field that attracts the happy or it promotes joy within its providers. I think it's probably both. One physician describes his perspective:

> I've never been a big Debbie Downer in general, so sure I have my days where things are upsetting and I get depressed, where I get sad by what the goings on are of the day, but my personality is such that I never let it... It never really sticks with me too long.
>
> It doesn't mean that I forget about the patients, stop thinking about them, or that I shut them off at the end of the day. I personally think the day that I do that or the day that I'm able to do that is the day I find another job because it means I've lost my humanity in this one. I think there is just a natural tendency for me to just sort of be on the more positive side than focus on the more negative stuff.

I managed to convince myself a long time ago that death is not the enemy. Pain and suffering are the enemy. I do have my spiritual and religious side. I don't know how much or to what extent that fits into this whole thing, but it is part of who I am.

You know, some days are just hard and there is no real thing that's going to change the fact that they're difficult. I don't make myself feel guilty for taking the time to not feel happy. I think the more you get yourself down about, why are you letting this affect you or whatnot? That just makes it so much worse for you.

What we do can be very heavy. What we do has its moments that are sad. You know what? I have to deal with that; but let me deal with it and then afterwards I'll get to a place where I'm not the Gloomy Gus.

What a beautiful idea, "Death is not the enemy. Pain and suffering are the enemy". I think if society and all of medicine really accepted this, many more patients would pass away with dignity and comfort. Our lives would be better. It is a simple concept, but contains so much meaning. The closing chapter of our life is defined in large part by the behavior and emotional composition of those around us. Patients, their families, and doctors act as emotional mirrors of each other. Each has the potential to orient his or her perspective towards a more positive direction. By doing so, one individual has the power to change the perspectives of peers and colleagues. Positive outlooks are contagious in pediatric oncology no matter the source, and the beauty in their prominence is most apparent near the end of life.

Doctors choose either consciously or unconsciously how emotionally invested they become with their patients, how close they get to the emotional fire so to speak. Some situations pull at their heartstrings because the patients remind them of their own children or the family is just so "nice". In treating patients of the same age as his own children, one doctor sees some advantages:

> I have a three-year-old girl. The three-year-old girls, the three or four-year-old girls that I see with Wilms' tumors, neuroblastoma, or leukemia, they're really hard. I mean, like you take care of them and you come home and see your kid running around and she is perfectly healthy. You can't help but wonder how you would react in that situation. I think that's why I give parents a lot of credit, and I try very hard to accommodate parents, because I can't even imagine what they go through on a daily basis. Forget during the initial diagnosis.
>
> I mean just what they go through on a daily basis, like their kid getting chemotherapy, their kid is sick. I can't even imagine what they go through, so yeah, I think that is a good way of

> putting it. I see my kid in them and I
> want them to get healthy and run around
> like my child does. And I see my child in
> them as well.

Other situations present themselves slowly and more explicitly; the doctor has a choice in how close to get to these families and patients. If the course is steadily progressing towards sadness either in treatment failure or eventual death, the doctor is able to engage at different personal and professional levels. The closer he or she gets, one could argue the more it will hurt when the outcome is bad.

So, I asked doctors what they practiced. How emotionally close did they get to their patients? Interestingly, about 85% of pediatric oncologists thought they got closer to their patients than their colleagues. This just isn't mathematically possible, but it's interesting nonetheless. Almost all of them used indicators of being on a first-name basis with parents and siblings of their patients, giving personal cell-phone numbers out to those near death, and knowing much about their patients' lives outside of the hospital. Most drew the line at social visits with families during active treatment or maintaining contact outside of a professional capacity. One doctor states:

> There are patients who are like, "You
> have to come to our house and we'll
> have breakfast." I don't do that kind of
> stuff. I'm not becoming their friend. I
> don't want to be their friend. I don't
> want to be involved in their personal life.

There are a couple parents whose kids have died who I'm friends with on Facebook or something. I keep in contact with them but I don't do anything like that while they're on therapy. There are very few patients who fall into that category and with whom I maintain that much contact.

But almost all had made exceptions to their "rules". They told me of families they had gone over to dinner at their houses, visited in far-off cities when traveling for other reasons, or even connected on Facebook. All said it was a rare occurrence, but the similarity was striking in each doctor's experience of breaking their customary emotional distance at least a couple times during their career. One had this to say on his overall approach:

> I don't think the way that most of us manage our emotional status is by not getting close to patients and families, that's only one way to deal with it. I think all of my colleagues, I believe, really become attached to the children and their parents. You spend so much time with them when they're going through this. Some of these families we may be seeing, on average, once or even more than once a week for years on end. I think that the reality is that most of the doctors, nurses, and nurse practitioners become close and attached to most of the families that we work with.

It's a little bit of a separate issue from, of course, how do you deal with the bad news the family may be receiving? How do you not let that affect you the same way that would affect the family? There, of course, I think it's important that you have some way that you deal with it.

Because if you were feeling the pain of every patient that you were taking care of, [nobody] could work in this field.

I think that, for me specifically, I guess I rely on the rational side of it to some degree. I try to see I've done everything possible to help the child, to help the family in every way. Not just with the treatment course, but including the palliative care they may need.

It could be with emotional support, or hooking them up with social services that they may need... or whatever it is. If I can feel, in the end, that I have done everything I could've possibly done and things go in a direction I wish it didn't go, I still may feel sad, but it's to a degree that I can handle and deal with.

Other doctors offered a different view. They maintained a more distant emotional relationship with patients and families. Some even thought that it allowed them to be more objective when approaching tough situations.

Here is one doctor reflecting on this approach:

> It depends a lot on personality, and I am not one of those who gets very close. I mean obviously there are some families that I get closer to and some families less. Although, I think each of us is able to dispense the same level of care to everyone. It is just... I don't know, maybe a client is similar to you or you relate to them more so you get a little bit closer... [for example] a kid who you may have more chemistry with than other kids.

> You kind of become close. I think at least for me the moment when things are going bad, then that is also the moment where I probably start that process of division.

> I never go to funerals. I think I went to two. I just don't, am not going to go, don't want to go anymore. Never going to go anymore. I don't like the wakes, and I really don't like the funerals. For me, I remember the child, when he was in the hospital or when he was outside the hospital in clinics. I remember when they don't survive or when I saw him or her dying in the hospital, but I don't like to go to wakes. Probably some families like to be part of that with the physician. Some families don't care if they are with

the physician because it is a family thing. I just don't like to go…

The reality is, at least for me, life goes on. This is the part of me that is at work, from which I learn a lot. I benefit a lot in terms of myself and my personality, but it is something that is part of me for a certain amount of time. I try not to make it spill into what is my family life, friend life, or anything else.

It remains with me and with my colleagues here, and I am sure it in some way transmits to my personality, my family life and things like that, but not in a direct way.

This honesty regarding her practice style was refreshing and also illuminating in her responses about funerals. While many pediatric oncologists do go to their patients' funerals, she clearly had her reasons for not going. Does that mean she doesn't care as much as the ones who do go? With a subtext of defensiveness, she explains that she doesn't like to go funerals of her deceased patients. I can see the validity in her points. These wakes and funerals can be filled with sadness and tears; attending one encourages a lasting mood around the event of contemplative sadness, reflection, and appreciation for the child lost.

But I more so think these events have the potential to be such demonstrations of beauty and celebrations of life. This notion is largely inspired by the wake and funeral I attended of a young boy who died from cancer. He passed away from acute myelogenous leukemia (AML) at age eight after a long journey, and we had grown close after being matched through a medical student program similar to Big Brothers Big Sisters. Remembering his wake and funeral, emotions flood back to me.

Walking into his wake, I was immediately struck by a collection of photos throughout the space. Each served as a reminder of his youthful, resilient spirit and the fact that he was just a child. There were baby pictures, kindergarten graduation photos, little league portraits, and family photos. His beaming smile and shining eyes lit up the page in every one. In only the way a photo of a child can do, they made me long for my own youth: the innocence, joy, and pure bliss. With each glimpse into his life, I then felt the aftershock's sting in realizing he was gone; there would be no more photos added to his album. Everywhere you looked on the shelves there were meticulously placed Star Wars Lego creations. He was an avid fan of Star Wars and Legos, and he took them apart and put them together even in the weeks leading up to his death. That room was compact, it was heavy, and milling about produced such a visceral feeling. Every vantage point reminded me of the beautiful life lost and shook my core in sadness. The focal point of that room and this memory is the open casket. It was smaller than any other casket I'd seen, and he looked so at peace—eyes shut with rosy cheeks, pale skin, and wispy hair—surrounded by his favorite stuffed animals.

The funeral was a similar onslaught of emotions. The entire nave was lit up in a rainbow of colors from the sunlight streaming through the stained glass. Listening to the father eulogizing his only son epitomized human anguish. At one point, they passed a microphone around and different friends and family shared thoughts they remembered. Little boys and girls told stories of playing together in the neighborhood; some were shy on the microphone and others babbled on in true childlike form. Most poignant was the mother; her voice radiated throughout the church as she told of her infinity of love. Her words faltered in moments of emotional breakdown and through all of the tears, her voice pierced all of us in that church. Listening to, watching, or hugging this mother at her son's funeral was an awe-inspiring experience. Feelings poured from her and filled that church. Amongst the sadness was also tremendous warmth. Remembering a child in a large group setting reminds us of the shared community a child creates. A child's funeral is incomparable; it is a moving experience that reinforces life's beauty and fleeting nature unlike any other.

As discussed before, the invitation to participate in and explore a family's sadness is a profound one; it is one of the most personal and vulnerable spaces in human existence. Watching parents and children work through and thrive in love despite sadness is so remarkable. It shows that strength and resilience are possible even in the most tragic of situations. There is an ebb and flow in cancer. It causes pain, and it causes tremendous sadness. But for the most part, children and families survive. About 80% of children with cancer are cured. So, although they will never forget the memories of very real sadness, they live long lives and have the chance to experience life's range of other emotions. In those families and children where the child passes away, yes, the sadness can seem unbearable at times. And yet, they cope despite sadness saturating their journeys. In fact, many find meaning and the full range of emotions including happiness even in those last months, weeks, or days. This continues after the child's death. In working through the aftermath, families and parents inspire us in their remarkable ability to identify their lasting love as supreme over their sadness. For one doctor, there were other emotions that dominate the experiences of families and patients with cancer:

> I think they would say hope. That's their first word. I think they would also say… I don't think sad. I think they would say anxious. I think they would say difficult, but I don't think most of them would say sad. I think they would say scary, but I think sadness is not a feeling that most of them have at the end. Rather, they experience it at points. I think sadness may be something that they feel about certain aspects of things… like things that could have been, but I think the overwhelming emotions are the ones that I have mentioned.

A mother and writer, Elizabeth Hall Hutner, beautifully talks about this feeling of love and gratitude for the time she had with her son, Sam, who lost his battle with cancer. Her response to others who tell her they understand her loss because they are also parents is, "No, now you understand what I had." This is an illustration of the immense strength in parents, something that not even cancer can break. Patients and families deal with sadness in many of the same ways doctors deal with sadness. They rationalize, find perspective, are supported by religion or spirituality, gain meaning from participating in research, and join support networks with other children and families. They definitely experience sadness, but with guidance and care are able to cope.

Yes, there are times when this sadness paralyzes parents and they feel defeated. From the blog posts of another mother, Ellyn Miller, who posts about her daughter, Gabriella, a little girl who died at age ten from brain cancer, we gain insight into the role of maternal instincts in cancer. She reflects:

> As a parent we want the best of and for our children. If they are hurt, we hurt even more. If they have achieved something that they are proud of, we are even more proud. Childhood cancer takes our ability to parent, knocks it to the ground, and stomps on it. It's neither like a cut that we can bandage nor like a cold or broken bone where you can take your child to a doctor to fix. Cancer renders us helpless.

Feeling helpless is one of the most dangerous feelings in medicine; it allows sadness to completely overwhelm. The solution is to find some way to feel empowered. This is not a one-time need because dealing with grief for parents who have lost a child is a never-ending journey. Another mother and blog poster, B.J. Karrer, who lost her son at age six, says, "Grieving the loss of a child is a process. It begins the day your child passes and ends the day the parent joins them." The online support group, Silent Grief, offers this similar thought:

> Grief from child loss is so tricky. It hides for a while, then when we least expect it, it seems to jump out of nowhere and grab us and not let go. Even while

driving along in the car just a certain "feeling" can overcome us and before we know it, we've pulled off to the side of the road and find ourselves openly weeping. The sadness inside of us escapes at the most unusual times making it so difficult for us. We just never know when the pain we feel inside is going to come out. This journey of child loss is the most uncharted, unpredictable journey we will ever travel. We never know from minute to minute what emotions will surface.

In life, emotional states tend to begin and end. We forgive and then are no longer bitter, we've moved on. We lose our feelings of anger to give way to acceptance. Happiness comes and goes. Yet, sadness does not recede with as much completeness. When introduced into a person's existence, sadness is a feeling that will linger indefinitely. It weaves throughout the rest of our lives, sometimes more present than others. Its occurrence fluctuates like other emotions, but it is unique in that it never completely disappears. It can always be tapped back into and felt with such intensity if accessed again. I think that is why it is difficult to characterize coping with sadness. For in pediatric oncology, to cope is not to vanquish sadness. It is neither an emotion that has a definite end nor one that has a universal approach in handling. Thus, in doctors, patients, and families, sadness is a feeling that must be learned to live alongside. This does not mean that those who feel sadness lead lives lost in an emotional fog. In many ways, a wise person can find more beauty and meaning in a life filled with sadness than another who lives blind to emotional perspective. Getting to that vantage point is the struggle.

During my five years of medical school, I've decided to treat children with cancer for the rest of my life as a pediatric oncologist. Some see my career decision as a choice to exist in such proximity to sadness and death. I choose to see it through other lenses. These children and families are the epitome of life. Each moment working with them is saturated in meaning, joy, and such raw emotional truth; that is the essence of life in all its glory. To find joy in helping to cure a child is easy. But to seek beauty and success in a child dying of cancer is harder but still possible. It is a task that I am ready for. I think in some ways it takes a strong person to stand beside the black hole of pediatric oncology. The environment is a constant vacuum; it is never satiated in time, emotions, or energy. At points in my future career, I know I will be closer than others to this black hole whether in sadness for my patients or exhaustion from my research. Sometimes I will be farther in it than others. But, I know I won't let it devour me. I will use perspective, hope, and fulfillment to crawl out of the black hole when I need it, to pull my patients and families out of it when they need it, and to ask others for help when I feel myself slipping deep inside. More importantly, patients and families will continue to remind us all that life in all its precious iterations is capable of magnificence.

CHAPTER 10

Happiness

"Never be sad for what is over, just be glad that it was once yours."

—Unknown

Happiness is a warmth. It is an emotion that saturates human thought with optimism and pleasure. Life speeds up in happiness; its direction whirls forward as if self-propelled with no impeding barriers. The whole world seems to bow to those who bask in happiness' glory. It is the siren to which we all long to be near. Those that find it are on top of the world. Yet, it taunts those who fail to find it. It beckons as a possibility to be achieved and remains as a mirage to some. To say happiness is a choice is a rebuke to those who fail to feel it, although this statement perhaps rings partly true. Happiness is not a pure emotion. Its greatest misconception is that it is the opposite of sadness. To look at them as polar opposites existing in complete separation is to overlook their intersection. Happiness exists in its own emotional sphere which grows in parallel along with sorrow. It remains happiness just the same, retaining all of its power because it occurs alongside sadness and not in spite of it. It is this thought which permeates pediatric oncology. Medicine is an assortment of emotions and not a tug of a war between opposing feelings. It is a collection of them all. That is what makes it truly beautiful. Doctors, families, and patients find happiness in the toughest of emotional situations. Children being cured of cancer or children dying of their disease, all of them can be versions of happiness.

As a medical student, my happiest times were unparalleled and ascended to an almost superhuman level; they always involved people or patients. For me, they were never a high-score on a test, an acceptance into a selective program, or a successful laboratory experiment. Happiness was always provoked by the smallest of moments and occurred when I, as a human, witnessed emotional realness in another person or family. A joyful father hearing his child was cured of cancer. A nurse dancing during a celebration commemorating a patient's last day of chemotherapy. Parents thanking me for explaining an illness in words and concepts they understood. Being told I was a patient's "favorite doctor" even though I wasn't yet a doctor. These situations engender simple happiness. I also experienced a more complex version of happiness in my training to this point. A mother hugs a daughter to soothe her after a blood draw or procedure. A father whispers, "I love you," to his sleeping child. A fellow medical student offers a kind message in a stressful time. A child faces cancer or death, experiencing it in their own brave way. Witnessing and participating in these events does not stir up the same simple happiness. This version of happiness is recognition of our shared humanity, the ephemeral condition of emotions, and life's magnificence in all of its permutations. Perhaps the ability to see happiness in this way was a conscious choice that I don't remember making. Perhaps it was more of an evolution. Or perhaps I was wired this way. For me, it is a beautiful way to view pediatric oncology and the larger world.

Doctors often find happiness when they find fulfillment. I believe it is this overlap that allows pediatric oncologists to remain so happy. Each of them is drawn to the opportunity to help children and families navigate an intense emotional journey. Many feel as if they are doing what they were born to do. Providers who chose to work with children with cancer find immense satisfaction. They find fulfillment in their careers, and through that fulfillment, find happiness. If the child is cured or if the child passes away, they still find this combination of fulfillment and happiness.

Patients that are cured provide doctors with much happiness. This is especially true when they've "beat the odds". Here is one doctor reflecting on one such case:

> I remember not ever thinking I would see this day, and now I do. She was seven when I met her. She's now eleven or twelve.
>
> She had a tumor from which she probably shouldn't have recovered, something called an ATRT, atypical teratoid rhabdoid tumor. We put her on a treatment... It's basically the kind of tumor where up until, I'd even say as much as ten years ago, every patient who was diagnosed with it usually died sometime around the one-year mark; but there had been a lot of work from a

couple of centers investigating chemotherapy strategies for them.

One of the hospitals that had really expended a lot of time and effort into this was [redacted], and I had been there, and I was comfortable with this protocol. So, when she came here and she was diagnosed, I put her on that.

After therapy, she was with no evidence of disease going in to surgery. She tolerated her surgery really well... She tolerated her treatment really well until her second to last course where she developed veno-occlusive disease of the liver and was in the PICU [the pediatric intensive care unit] and almost died. She is this little girl. Her parents are both [Eastern European]. They're both dentists. I have [Eastern European] family. It's a disease that I really hate, and so I really want to win over that disease, but I also just fell in love with this family, and I fell in love with the little girl, and she survived that episode.

We made the decision to give her no more chemotherapy, and in October or December, we are doing her three-years-out-of-treatment scan. Actually, it'll be three and a half years. I remember not ever thinking I would see this day and I do now.

Curative stories produce happiness for all involved. There are typically many other emotions along the way, but being part of a team that has cured a child with cancer generates an unmatched level of pure happiness. These children and families persevere through a roller coaster of intense and sometimes unexpected emotions, but reaching a cure results in a sense of bliss that overcomes all else. A pediatric oncologist remembered:

> There are all sorts of contenders for my favorite patient, or the most dramatic patient, or something like that. I think probably if you asked me this question ten times, I'd give you ten different answers. One patient who is really close to my mind is a family that I met when we first started taking care of their little girl. The story goes back even further because her father was a survivor of retinoblastoma. I did not care for him, but then when he and his wife were having their first child, they knew that the little girl had inherited the RV1 mutation from him. We met the child when she was a neonate. I think, actually at the beginning she didn't even have retinoblastoma in her eyes, but we followed her closely. She developed retinoblastoma early in life, and her eyes were cured with laser therapy only, so this was a great success. She didn't need radiation or chemotherapy.

Everything was good until about her second birthday, when she presented to the ER [emergency room] with signs of increased intracranial pressure. She was found to have a rare version of retinoblastoma called trilateral retinoblastoma when, in addition to having tumors in both eyes, she had a pineal gland tumor. At the time that this was recognized in her, this was thought to be a 100% fatal condition. There were very rare cases that had been reported where children had survived, but all of those had been when the child presented asymptomatically, where a tiny tumor was found on a screening scan.

So, this was pretty bad. Her parents were very intelligent. The dad is in the financial field. The mom is a lawyer. The grandfather is actually a pathologist who had done a lot of work in this field. So, we had long discussions with them and explained that this was very high risk, but we had treated children with malignant brain tumors that were related with very intensive chemotherapy. We'd had some promising results. We thought it was worth trying to treat this little girl hopefully.

So, we treated her with intensive chemotherapy and second look surgery. At the end of the treatment, with her very high dose chemotherapy, she was as close to dying from complications as any patient that I've taken care of. Somehow she pulled through this and she survived and came back out of the intensive care unit, and as time passed and the disease didn't take her, I started to become optimistic that maybe this was going to have a happy ending tumor-wise, and maybe she was going to be cured.

But, she had had a big brain tumor. She'd had hydrocephalus. She'd had neurosurgery. She'd been in the intensive care unit on a ventilator for a long time. So, I was still pretty worried about... although we hadn't given her brain radiation, what were the consequences of all this really going to be? And thinking we had cured her but maybe she was going to be developmentally delayed.

Then, when she was a little bit older, she would come into clinic with her father, and her father would start telling me what had happened since the last visit, and the little girl would start correcting him. She'd say, "That's not correct, it happened this other way." And he'd say [to her], "Yeah, you're right."

And as time went on, of course she went to school and things. She is a good student in school, so beyond the fact that she was cured of what seemed like an invariably lethal disease, I realized that thankfully all these problems had not unduly taken a toll on her directed memory and things like that. She seems very likely to live a normal quality of life, despite everything. To me, that's certainly high on my list of rewarding patient stories.

And here is another. This story links fulfillment, tragedy, happiness, success, and gratitude. It blurs the lines connecting each emotion, bringing them to the same level:

I'll just tell you about her because she is a survivor. This was a little girl who I took care of during fellowship [at an East Coast hospital]. She was a little under two when she was diagnosed. She had stage III neuroblastoma. I picked her up halfway through my fellowship. She had high risk disease because she had Myc-N amplified tumor. So, she got very intensive chemotherapy and bone marrow transplant surgery, the whole sorta nine yards.

At the end of fellowship, I moved to [a city on the West Coast] to get a job and the family said, "Well we're going to come with you." At that point, she was in follow-up and in complete remission. They had moved back to [the Caribbean island where they lived]. They were going to come to [the hospital on the East Coast] every three months to see me, and they said, "Well we're just going to come to [the West Coast] every three months. If we have to fly somewhere, you're her doctor; we're going to fly to see you." So, this was a huge compliment. Because she was from [a Caribbean island], they didn't have the resources to take care of her there. Her dad had gone to school [in a city on the East Coast] and knew people [in that city].

They immediately came to [East Coast city] when she was diagnosed and then the mom basically moved into the Ronald McDonald house for six months of the treatment, six months plus. We just became very close. The little girl was spunky and very strong willed. At the time she was an only child and she was really sick; but I just really liked her spirit. She just was very spunky. Her family was lovely and they just were really terrific. It's been two years since I've seen her and in the intervening two years, they had another baby.

The father was in a very serious car accident and was in a coma for over a month and has made what sounds like a full recovery. She's coming to see me next week for her... she's six plus years from diagnosis and her likelihood of relapse should be extremely low. They're the one family where I have had a social meal with them. I never, ever do it but I went to a wedding in [the island where they live] and I said, "Well I have to see them." So, we went out for dinner. When they came here in the past, I've taken them out for lunch. Just because they're coming all this way, I have to see them outside of the hospital.

Now she's eight. Her dad has always said, "In Latino culture, there's the fifteenth birthday, the quinceañera, they have a big birthday party and he's from day one has said, "You are going to come to her fifteenth birthday party on the beach." Now I really think it's going to happen because she's so far out from her treatment. Knock on wood she doesn't get a secondary malignancy; she's likely going to be a long-term survivor. That would be very gratifying. She's definitely a favorite and everyone knows she's my favorite.

To be able to tell families and children that the cancer has been cured is a feeling unmatched in medicine and perhaps life in general. Giving families the news of a cure propels emotions into the stratosphere and provides much motivation for providers in stark contrast to the stereotype of the field as one filled with sadness. 80% of children with cancer are cured and many more will survive with chronic treatment and lead productive, long lives. The conversation at the end of treatment, the one families have been hoping, dreaming, and praying for since the diagnosis was made, is almost always led by the doctor. When the doctor is sharing the news that the cancer is cured, it is an encounter which can only be described as a true celebration:

> Yeah. As soon as someone hears pediatric oncology they say, "Oh God, that's so hard. That must be so hard." I actually have never felt that it is that hard. I really enjoy it. While it is painful to see the families going through this, I think that part of being an oncologist not only do you get to give parents this horrible news but you also then… Just yesterday, I got to call up a family and say, "Great news. I just got MRD [minimal residual disease] back after induction. He's officially in remission. We can't detect leukemia." Eight weeks ago I was giving them the worst news of their life and now suddenly I get to turn around and give them the best news of their life.

> In general pediatrics they're never getting to tell patients and families the best news of their life. It's a huge swing.

Even when a child is not cured and dies, there is still happiness to be found in this heart-breaking situation. There is much joy even in dying children. Providers find this through their experiences in helping families and children accomplish goals, have comfortable journeys, and create meaningful experiences in the last months and weeks. They focus on quality of life and develop a perspective that values each moment. Here is one doctor describing a patient on his way toward an expected death. This is never the outcome anyone wishes for, yet it is a story filled with life. When asked about his favorite patient, this was the doctor's response:

> There isn't one. I'm looking at the mural over there. He's the one I'm thinking about now, see the guy kicking the soccer ball?
>
> He is a little miracle and he's also a genius. He is about ten years old and he has neuroblastoma from here to here [*he motions from head to toe*]. The simple answer is that I have a new favorite patient every... It depends on when you ask, who I see in clinic. I love all of them. There are some that get under your skin. He is something else. He's kicking that soccer ball with tumor literally all through his body... he was going to die.
>
> Then he went on a phase I study and he was on that for forty-seven months, still able to play soccer through it. Now, he's home on basically palliative care, he's on palliative chemotherapy. That was a hard discussion that we just had a week or so ago with the family, getting them to realize the time's running out. He's had

everything over ten times; the tumor
continues to march on.

I talked to mom on Monday and they're
at some cabin in the woods enjoying the
lake. He was pain free and doing okay.

The simple answer is that there's a new
patient everyday that's a favorite.

The above situation is universally difficult and embodies
many emotions including sadness, but also hope, comfort,
and happiness. It is possible to see these moments of being
"pain free" and feeling "okay" as significant, happy
accomplishments in a dying child. The key is to find
perspective and place value in quality of life rather than
length. New personal growth and beautiful experiences do
not stop occurring once families find out their child is dying.
In fact, it becomes more important for them to recognize
where to look and how to create them. Doctors are
experienced in finding that fulfillment and thus are well-
positioned to lead families and children with cancer towards
that same emotional vantage point.

To bring families and children closer to finding
happiness throughout their cancer journeys, doctors must
form very close, trusting relationships. It is these same
relationships that are most significant to the doctors. It is
these relationships that keep them happy. In characterizing
the field, one says:

I love what I do, and I've always wanted
to do it. It's actually a lot more hopeful
than people think. I usually tell them that

> most pediatric oncology patients survive their cancer, as opposed to adults. I get to have these really awesome relationships with families and patients. I enjoy having those relationships; they are very fulfilling for me.

These caring relationships between providers, families, and patients motivate the doctors to continue to work in the field of oncology.

> I would say I feel like I've been able to make a difference. I also feel—it's kind of an odd thing—selfish isn't the right word, self-serving isn't the right word. It's odd to me that I can feel so fulfilled with, it's a very, the human to human connection to me is very fulfilling. So every day I have the opportunity to connect with human beings and share in the honor of such intimate life experiences... I'm happy. I am pleased that I found a profession that I can be successful at and make a living at. At the end of the day, I feel like what I've done has truly made a difference and I think that's why I like it... I don't want to give up; I want to help these kids live and I totally get it.

To live in the moment, no matter what context that moment is in, is one of the strongest ways to encourage happiness. If that moment occurs at a ten-year-cancer-free party, great, celebrate it with joy. But if that moment occurs in the hospital with a child who has relapsed with his cancer and is dying, celebrate it just the same. This sentiment is essentially mindfulness, a meditational practice focused on experiencing the present moment, its thoughts, and feelings without judgment. Mindfulness is a powerful way to feel and identify happiness in the present moment and shift emotions as one physician expressed:

> There's this one kid I think of who wasn't even my primary patient, but I just became very close to the family because he was just such a sweet and wonderful young man. We eventually lost him, and that was hard on me. He's the kind of guy... He was the sort of patient who would have me paged and is like, "Doctor, you said we were going to go play Scrabble." I'm like, "You know what? You're right, I did. We're going to." No matter what I was doing, what deadlines I had, it was just like, "Pfft, no. He wants to play Scrabble, and we're doing it." He had Ewing's sarcoma. He was twenty-five when he passed away.

In these above stories and in each provider's quotes in this book, it is evident that happiness is present throughout pediatric oncology. While it may not be the typical depiction of a toddler smiling with an ice cream cone on the beach, it is happiness just the same. It does not occur only when everything aligns in joyful harmony with a fairytale's "happily ever after". Happiness charges through rough times as a ray of hope, an unstoppable laugh, or a candid smile. It refuses to be silenced once given the opportunity to reveal itself. Children create so much happiness in this world, with or without cancer. A smile is a smile; a laugh is a laugh, and each conveys the full power and contagion of this emotion. In my interviews with pediatric oncologists across the United States, I asked many doctors to tell me stories of their favorite patients. Below is one that touched me most about a remarkable boy with a brain tumor:

> I have a patient right now who is really neat. He is a fourteen-year-old kid coming from [a Caribbean island], and he speaks almost no English. He has a big low grade glioma [a type of brain tumor], it's huge. He should have been diagnosed about seven years ago but because he's in a third world country, it's been growing for years, since forever.
>
> He comes in here and this is the first time I met him. At the end of our conversation he says, "Doctor, where are the sick children of [the hospital]?" I said, "Julio [a pseudonym], I don't understand, what do you mean?" I'm talking to him in Spanish. I'm like, "Really, I don't understand what you mean." And he says again, "Where are the sick children of [the hospital]?" Mind you, this is one of the sick kids of [the hospital]. So, I said, "Well Julio, there are some patients upstairs in the hospital and there are others in the housing."

He goes, "Great, because I want to play my guitar for them and sing for them and put smiles on their faces." This is a kid who just got here for his newly diagnosed brain tumor who wants to go put smiles on other kids' faces.

So, this is kind of what ends up happening to me. These are the kids I'm most drawn to or find myself really enjoying spending time with. These kids who think outside themselves, that rise above in the midst of a really bad situation. They are so able to bring a smile to my face.

Children with cancer have a beautiful ability to create happiness. In both the triumphs and struggles of their lives, they provide inspiration as a gift to the doctors, families, and other children who have the privilege of being part of their journeys.

As a multidimensional emotion, happiness is a shape-shifter of sorts. It easily sprouts from feelings of fulfillment, hope, faith, and trust. But, it can also launch from sadness, fear, shock, and anger. Its relationship with these other emotions is convoluted and complex. It takes conscious thought and determination to recognize happiness in sadness, but it is possible. Doctors, patients, and families have found immense meaning and fulfillment in a broad spectrum of emotional experiences throughout pediatric oncology. These experiences range from a child who is cured of cancer to a child who passes away from the disease. In each, there are strong themes of happiness. Transforming or broadening an emotional experience from one defined by sadness to one marked by happiness is a beautiful process. It provides incredible meaning to pediatric oncology and life in general. I am learning this practice and seeing the world in a more positive light.

Afterword

"Children with cancer are like candles in the wind who accept the possibility that they are in danger of being extinguished by a gust of wind from nowhere and yet, as they flicker and dance to remain alive, their brilliance challenges the darkness and dazzles those of us who watch their light."

—Unknown

E motions are real. They are beautiful. They deserve consideration. Emotions define and shape all experiences. The happenings of a moment, a day, or even a life mean little to us without the feelings that permeated those events. As emotions are the metric to judge an experience, their occurrences merit attention. To live a meaningful life is to examine our experiences and parse out the milieu of feelings in ourselves and in those around us. All human beings should do this including doctors, patients, families, medical students, nurses, and other providers. In doing so, we can lead more full, rich lives and inspire others to do the same. To understand our emotions, we need to reflect on the unique personal context and history of our emotions but also the setting in which they occurred. Emotions do not occur in vacuums or in only one person at a specific time. They are never solitary undertakings even if we make attempts to isolate or conceal their development or manifestations. Feelings are strengthened or dampened as they intersect with the feelings of others who share in the experience. Sadness takes on a different quality when it is shared in the presence of others. Happiness expands if allowed to pool with neighboring joy. Fear, anger, hope, trust, shock, and faith all transform if they occur in proximity to other individuals experiencing similar or even different emotions. To steer an experience or a life towards more fulfillment and satisfaction on an emotional level requires reflection from multiple viewpoints. It is important to consider personal feelings, but also the emotional responses your actions and even feelings summon in those around you. Emotions are one of the most human conceptions. They are eternal ideas. They deserve reverence and thought from all angles.

This book is an emotional exploration of the field of pediatric oncology. The perspectives include those of doctors, medical students, families, and children with cancer from a personal, clinical, and intellectual level; these were elicited through a number of interviews at multiple hospital sites in the United States. All of the feelings discussed are not unique to pediatric oncology; they are universal human emotions. All of us have dealt with them to a varying degree. While the emotional threads in this book are tethered to pediatric oncology, non-medical readers can make connections with their own lives.

The capacity to feel makes us human. It should be the basis of our relationships, define our communities, and be one of the major motivations in our lives. The road to understanding your emotions is the most personal and challenging journey to embark on. Do not do it alone. Emotions are a collective experience; understanding them to further maximize their utility should be too. So, talk about them. Think about them. Feel them. The modern world is one which emotional subtleties are glossed over for the convenience of expediency, politeness, lack of openness, or fear of dismissal. Do not dull yourself and gray your emotional range.

I hope you also take from this book that children with cancer are not defined by one emotional dimension of sadness. The oncologists I worked with and interviewed did not think so. The families in reflecting on their journeys did not think so, and the actual children themselves were filled, on the contrary, with a mature sense of hope, resilience, and happiness. This is not to say there aren't currents of sorrow, but to cast the field and those with cancer as sad is to characterize an existence without recognizing that sadness is but one theme in their lives and those who work with these children. The challenges are difficult and the disease is brutal, but these children embody and inspire life in those who have the privilege to share in their journeys. More than their sadness, their spirited resilience spreads to those who love and work with them.

It is worth remembering that life is defined by its depth and not its length. The range of experiences and memories—the good, the bad, the love, the anger, and the sadness—constitute an existence. This is true in everyone and especially in children with cancer. To judge the life of a child who dies from cancer as "too short" is to miss one of this book's central themes. That thought process focuses the discussion on the number of days of heartbeats rather than the richness and range of a unique life.

Many people are inspired by children with cancer to "remember that life can be over at any second", to "be grateful for your health", or that "life is unfair". I don't completely disagree with these sentiments, but I feel that children with cancer should most inspire us to value life's vitality and emotional range. Life is not fragile because it is possible for cancer to cut it short. Life is most fragile because each moment presents a choice to allow feelings to rise in us and be experienced or to not. It is a choice between living with true emotions and living with a blunted version letting time pass us by. In many moments, this choice may seem minor or inconsequential having no rippling effects. Yet, I posit that these moments build. This is the delicate nature of emotions and life. Each time we curtail or dismiss our feelings, we chip away a sliver from our expressive being. We become less able to share in the many forms of life in all its beauty because we have become less accustomed to talking and thinking about them. So, I most urge you to use this book, its stories, and perspectives as a place to begin.

"To laugh often and much; to win the respect of intelligent people and the affection of children; to earn the appreciation of honest critics and endure the betrayal of false friends; to appreciate beauty; to find the best in others; to leave the world a bit better whether by a healthy child, a garden patch, a redeemed social condition; to know even one life has breathed easier because you lived. This is to have succeeded."

—Ralph Waldo Emerson

Acknowledgments

The world of medicine owes tremendous gratitude to its patients, as does this book. I'd like to thank all of the children with cancer and their families for sharing their lives and stories. This book would not have been possible without all of the support staff who coordinated my hospital site visits and doctors who graciously let me follow them around with a clipboard in hand and sat down with me to be interviewed. I am grateful for their insight, anecdotes, and warm invitations to converse at length about a deeply personal topic: emotions. This beautiful experience and their words have and will continue to shape my perspectives in life and medicine.

For literary support and encouragement, I give tremendous thanks to Dr. Stephanie Brown Clark who served as my primary advisor and editor for this book, all along providing thoughtful guidance in an inspirational manner. For the chance to live a year as a writer, an opportunity of a lifetime considering I spent much of it in Barcelona writing under the shadow of the Sagrada Familia, I am indebted to The Division of Medical Humanities and Bioethics at the University of Rochester. I am so grateful to have received a grant and logistical support to bring my project to fruition. In addition, I'd like to thank Drs. David

Korones, OJ Sahler, and Jeffrey Andolina for being mentors in this project and model physicians to emulate as I move forward with my career.

To the University of Rochester medical student community past and present for editing selections of my book, thank you for reminding me that our school is a remarkable and special place where fellow students are eager to help one another. Those benevolent individuals include: David Valentine, Michelle Pitch, Anna Jaffe, Zehui Wang, Dr. Peter Capucilli, Jonathan Lin, Dr. Margaret Compton, Rachel Cameron, Bryan Brown, Graham Bevan, Jason Lyou, Jennifer Luong, Melissa Hewson, Lam-Anh Nguyen, Benjamin Cocanougher, James Bates, Trevor Hansen, William Archibald, Dr. Sabina Khan, Kimberley Thoms, Mark Miller, Nan Zhu, Nicholas Reiter, and Ryen Alicandro.

Finally, I'd like to thank my loving family who has helped me to get where I am now and to be confidently excited about my future. This includes my mom, Monica, who radiates positivity about life and encourages my friendly nature in seeing the best in people. To my dad, Tim, I always feel supported by you and it pushes me to be a better, stronger person as I seek to live up to your example. For my siblings, Kelly, Nick, and Tim, thank you for being my three best friends and for the lifetimes of experiences that we've had as we've grown older. And to my grandmother, Jean, who reminded me to finish this book by often inquiring about its status in a gentle, caring way that only a grandma is capable of, you are an inspiration. May one day I build a family as emotionally connected and loving as the one you have created. That would be quite the life.

63620766R00119

Made in the USA
Lexington, KY
12 May 2017